Reclaim Your Health

*Permanent Weight Loss and
Simple Steps to Nutritional Literacy*

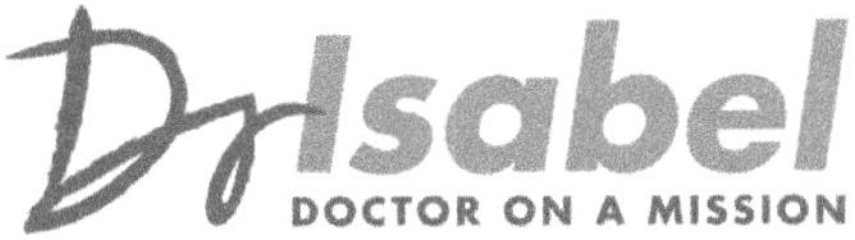

Contents

Introduction

"If you don't like it, change it."
–Unknown

I HAVE BEEN A DOCTOR since 1991. The only reason I went into the medical field was because I wanted to help people. Looking at what is going on in medicine today, I have come to the realisation that we don't have a healthcare system – we only have Disease Management. Not only did I become disillusioned and burnt out, I just got frustrated treating conditions rather than the causes of problems.

I wanted to get to the root of the dis-ease, not just throw a band-aid on it. My patients weren't getting any better, they were just existing. My goal is to see people healed.

Hence the reason for the above quotation: "If you don't like it, change it." I had to change the way I was doing medicine, and let me say: It's not easy. But I knew I had to do it, both for the people I care for, and for my sanity.

Over the last decade I began to learn about nutrition, exercise and lifestyle choices to help you live a more healthy life. Yes, I want to help you make a positive change in your life. My goal is to add value to your life by offering you simple backpocket principles which you can use every day.

If you want to lose weight permanently, have more energy and infect the lives of your family and friends with health, then I invite you to *Reclaim Your Health*.

Congratulations on purchasing *Reclaim Your Health!*

Becoming a Registered Reader

Over the next few years we will be experiencing a revolution in Medicine, where everyone will be given the tools for better health, and not have to live with chronic un-wellness. We are all invited to take part.

Because you have invested in your health by purchasing this book, we would like to keep you up-to-date with the latest nutritional information. We would love to have you join the team by signing up for our FREE newsletter at:

www.doctoronamission.com

> *Check **www.doctoronamission.com**
> for the dates of our upcoming
> **14-DAY WEIGHT LOSS COURSE:**
> your start to permanent weight loss.*

Dedication

I WANT TO DEDICATE this book to two very special people in my life.

To Mima (aka Mom, Silvia): Your beautiful love and faith in me I will never, ever forget.

To my husband, Michael: Your devoted love, patience, and maximising friendship steered me while I said, "Let's go this way."

"Within every patient there resides a doctor,
and we as physicians are at our best
when we put our patients in touch
with the doctor inside themselves."
– Albert Schweitzer M.D.

Success Stories

Attending *Reclaim Your Health Workshop* gave Murray and me the impetus to make several big but necessary changes to our lifestyle. The course was presented in a fun, interactive way and gave us the motivation to make some healthy changes. Before attending the course we had often talked about making some changes, but had never got around to it or even figured out where to start. Since doing the course we have built regular exercise routine and big changes in our eating habits. Thanks Mike and Izzy! We would definitely recommend this course to anyone who is thinking they could do with a healthier lifestyle. The benefits are well worth it.

– Murray and Vicki Crozier

I chose to take part in *Reclaim Your Health Workshop* for a number of reasons, but most of all because I knew the way I was living, eating and thinking was not going to see me through life in good health. After all, takeaways and rubbish food are so convenient, not to mention life is so busy that we all forget that we still need to find a balance.

Throughout the course I was blessed to be given the tools that would not only see me through life as a healthy individual, but also enable me to hand down those tools to family, friends and the wider community. These tools include healthy cooking and eating, which foods are going to cause illness and damage to my precious body, how to exercise without having the excuse of "I don't have time", as well as how important it is to have a happy healthy brain that can plant positive seeds to grow a positive person.

Since completing the course my health and outlook on life have completely changed, with such awesome results! Thanks to the tools *Reclaim Your Health Workshop* provided me with, we as a family now live a healthy, active and fun-filled life, and not once has it been a struggle to implement this into our day-to-day living. I cannot thank Mike and Izzy enough for saving me and my family from the convenience and fuss of today's busy lifestyles. Mike and Dr. Izzy, you guys rock. Thanks.

– Nita Gaylord

Earlier this year three of my children and I attended the *Reclaim Your Health* programme. Michael and Dr. Isabel Hunsinger presented an extremely enjoyable and informative programme. This couple are truly passionate and knowledgeable about health and living a healthy lifestyle. Michael being an experienced executive chef and Isabel a doctor, you could not ask for better teachers to deliver this life-changing programme.

I learned so much from Isabel about how the body works: why we feel tired after eating certain foods; hungry not long after we have just eaten; the good foods we can eat that give us energy and keep us full for longer. One of the things I enjoyed best was learning how to lose weight without that nasty four-letter word 'DIET'. Eat, don't go hungry, and lose weight. How the body works, why it does what it does and why your energy levels feel the way they do, was amazing to learn. The way Isabel presented the information made it fun and easy to learn. You can feel her passion.

Once we learned about the different foods we had a cooking night with Executive Chef Mike. "WOW, PRICELESS" are two words I have to say about what I came away with that night. Mike made it so easy to make a healthy meal and incorporate 9–12 different coloured fruits and vegetables. I am a mother who works a full time career. I used to always stress over what to make for dinner in a timely manner, so the children would still get to bed on time.

Mike showed us how to spend a couple of hours once a week cutting up veg-es, then how to keep them fresh in the refrigerator. Prepare your meat for the week. Open your fridge and everything is there that you need to cook healthy meals for the week. I now know how to make healthy meals for my family in a small amount of time. That for me is priceless. I just want to thank Chef Michael and Dr. Isabel from the bottom of my heart for putting together such an amazing, life-changing programme. I have learned so much, and for that I thank you.

– Heather Valdez

My Story

I was born on December 26 1959 in Washington DC. Now I don't tell everyone my birthday – but because you have decided to read this, I thought it best that you get to know who I am from the beginning.

The decision to become a doctor was planted in my mind when I was five years old. My uncle Dr. Julio Perez, an anaesthesiologist, has this amazing way about him. When he walked into the room his smile, his positive attitude, would light up the room. He would just make you feel happy, and you would start smiling. At five years of age I decided, and said to my mom, "I want to be a doctor like Tio Julito" (Uncle Julio in Spanish).

At 18, after graduating from high school, I was looking through a *Mother Earth* magazine and saw that there was an organic farm in Pennsylvania that needed help. A few weeks later I was working at the Lefevers Organic Farm in Spring Grove. That was an eye-opening experience. Not only did I learn how to grow our own sprouts on the windowsill of the kitchen, but I was also exposed to mulching, running a health food shop, and organic farming.

Winter came and there was no work at the farm, and I was referred to two ladies who were opening a health food restaurant in York Pa., called The Sproutery. Paula and Cindy were really into fresh vegetable juices and I was the Juicer Girl. We were juicing wheatgrass, carrot, celery and beetroot by the glass. It was new, fun, and exciting.

In 1979 I decided it was time to get serious and go to college. After all the exposure to organic farming and eating, I naturally decided to major in Agriculture and become an organic farmer. I thought Colorado would be a good place, so I applied to Colorado State University (CSU), got an interview, and hopped on a bus with my three-litre bottle of organic apple juice and fasted the whole way (three days to be exact) until I was deposited at the Fort Collins, Colorado, bus depot.

The acceptance letter came in the mail, and I was off to CSU to become an organic farmer. There was just one little problem I encountered in my first year of college … I soon realised that plants don't talk to you, and I'm a very social being. So, I decided again that I was going to become a doctor.

I withdrew from Agriculture and headed to Boulder Colorado to start my new major, this time as a pre-med student in Molecular Cellular Developmental Biology. I absolutely loved-loved-loved this major, because it taught me how everything works from the DNA level all the way to the completed picture of the human being.

During the middle of the four-year degree I was having thoughts of becoming a naturopath. The rationale was it was more holistic, and I would learn about taking care of the root of the disease. I really wanted to take care of people without drugs.

I mentioned this to my anatomy professor Dr. Tom Swain. He shook his head, smiled that gorgeous smile he always had, and recommended that I go the MD way. His philosophy was, you can make more change in medicine once you are on the inside as an MD. He knew I was already unhappy with the medical system's lack of treatment of the root cause of the disease, instead treating it with medication. I wasn't even a doctor yet, I was still in pre-med … but I knew I needed to become a doctor of medicine.

There are times in my life when I become pensive and wonder what my life would have been like if I had become rebellious and prideful and not taken Dr. Swain's advice. To this date I am so grateful he cared enough to mentor me into medicine. Thank you Tom!

I made it through medical school and found it very unfair and cutthroat. The amount of minutiae we had to memorise seemed – and still seems – pointless. The whole system would benefit from an overhaul.

After 22 years of being a doctor now, I have seen my patients become more unwell and more overweight. They just aren't getting any better. So over the last 10 years I have been studying Functional Medicine, which focuses on the root cause of disease and its treatments. One passion of mine is weight loss, because I know how distressful even an extra 2.2 kg (five pounds) can be, let alone 45 kgs (100 pounds)!

Let me give you an overview of my previous health. During my medical training, a typical breakfast was candy and coffee. Then throughout the day, just to stay awake, I would have at least six cups of coffee. When there was time I would eat a meal. Then when work was done and I didn't have to sleep in the hospital, I would go home.

To me five o'clock meant wine o'clock, and I would have a glass or two to wind down from all the caffeine. Not only was I hooked on caffeine and sugar, but also a nighttime wine to wind down.

I also partook in cigarette smoking. Yes, I was a model of health. It took me 41 times to quit smoking…but I finally did it. From that comes my motto to my patients: "Never, ever, ever give up giving up!"

When I gave birth to my second child I weighed in to the hospital at 90 kg (198 pounds) and came out at 189 pounds. I am only five feet six inches (166cm)! It took me 16 years to get down to 73 kg (160 pounds), and I did every diet possible except take diet pills. I was deeeeeesperate. Now over the last two years, from all my studying, I am 61 kg (135 lbs) and 53 years young. I am so excited to share with you how to get rid of excess weight safely – and keep it off. My conversion to the other side of the medical spectrum happened gradually, and hit its stride when I had my 50th birthday. I just realised that I really wanted to be healthy and walk my talk.

And so here we are together. Let's start walking together, and I'll share with you what worked for me and can also work for you. I want to give you hope.

Your friend,

Dr. Isabel

> *"Hope is not pretending that problems don't*
> *exist. It is the hope that they don't last forever.*
> *That hurts will heal and difficulties be overcome.*
> *That we will be led out of the darkness*
> *and into the light."*
> –The Optimism Revolution

CHAPTER ONE

Your Metabolism and Nutrition
People are destroyed by lack of knowledge

1. The Circle of Change...ouch!

Why do we do what we do, when we know what we know?

That is the question we need to ask ourselves when we are deciding to make a change. For instance, we know smoking is not good for our health, yet people continue to smoke. Yes it has to do with the addiction, but it also has a lot to do with the circle of change.

The circle of change pertains to the doors we go through as we are changing. No one likes to change. It feels uncomfortable. We have set habits in place and even if they are killing us, they are familiar to us. They bring a sense of stability to our lives.

There are two basic human tendencies: we either avoid pain or seek pleasure. Which one do you think wins? Yes, you are right...avoidance of pain. We will do anything to avoid pain.

The avoidance of pain is why everyone, including me, wants a quick fix – a quick fix to weight loss. The reality is, there will never be a quick fix. There is no such thing as microwaveable health. We have to put in the work to get the results. The cool thing is that what you will learn here in Your PureLifestyle Plan is how to create new, healthy habits that will keep the weight off.

You will create a New Normal for yourself. And when you fall off track, as we all do, you will notice that you feel wrong. Heather Valdez, one of my clients in New Zealand, says it best: "When I fall off track and start eating the wrong foods

…I feel dirty and want to get clean again." That is exactly the point. Heather has created a New Normal for herself, and it is comfortable for her.

Let's take a look at the phases you go through to create change.

Phase 1. Pre-Contemplation

This is called the waiting game. The door is shut tight. For me as a healthcare worker, this is the most frustrating stage. Why? Because I'm waiting for people either to wake up or just be pushed into having to change their situation.

For instance, imagine it's 8am in the morning and you are getting ready for work, and on the way to work, bam! – you start having chest pain. Next you are in the Emergency Department being told you are having a heart attack. This could be the time you are pushed into doing something about your health … or maybe not.

However, if you do start to think about making some lifestyle change, then you are moving into the next phase.

Phase 2. Contemplation

The door is slightly ajar. This is when you are thinking about making a change. It is here you start to build your confidence. You are looking at ways to "make the change" as Michael Jackson says.

Phase 3. Preparation

I love this phase because the door is open and it's time for intervention. You are teachable and motivated.

Phase 4. Action and Maintenance Stage

Here you are managing your craving by controlling your challenging thoughts. When problems arise you have a plan of attack.

Phase 5a. The goal is reached

Here you either reset a new goal or stay at your new level for normal.

OR

Phase 5b. The relapse

And we are back at phase 1. This is where we wait for phase 2 to begin.

So now you know why people do what they do, when they know what they know. It all goes back to where they are in the circle of change.

I trust you are all in phase 3. And for reaching this phase, let me be the first to tell you today (if no one has beat me to it already), that you are a radiant being!

I cannot change you – or anyone. You come to this stage all on your own. In the past I used to push people to this stage and it was like pushing a parked car uphill. Nothing happened.

I learned a long time ago that you can lead a horse to water. but if that horse doesn't want to drink…guess what? It won't.

If you change and achieve your goal because of something I taught you, then all the applause goes to you. You have made the decision to change and implement what you've learned. I didn't change you, you did. You made the decision for a better life with better health. You own that power, not me. Yes, you truly are a radiant being!

Writing Down Your Goals

Studies have shown that people who write down their goals have a higher rate of achievement than people who don't. Writing them down begins the launch, and the next step appears. If you don't, then the next execution step never arrives.

"But what if I don't reach my goal?"

That's a fantastic question. No big deal – you reset it. At least you've started moving forward and up.

Before we go any further, as your health coach, I ask you to write down answers to the following questions:

1. What is your health goal?

2. Why do you care about your health?

For me, I have pictures of my family in my mind. They need me to be my best for the journey. My husband Michael says "Happy wife, happy life." That's certainly true, and I have a responsibility to do my part to be a happy wife, mother, doctor, friend.

I also think of my goals in life. In particular, my goal in medicine is to coach more than a million health workers around the world to go into schools, businesses, families, places of worship to help people reclaim their health, both mentally and physically.

3. What would stop or deter you from reaching your goal?

Is it your family, friends, workmates? It's good to know where the bumps in the road will be so you can be prepared.

4. Who is on your support team?

TEAM stands for Together Everyone Achieves More. You know *I'm* on your team, but who else? *You* need to be on your team and be kind to yourself when you are talking to yourself.

Remember that what you conceive, you can achieve. By writing your goals down you are conceiving. I encourage you to take the time to invest in yourself by writing #1–4 down.

Now that you have that completed, we can go onto the next step.

2. Blood Sugars

What we eat and when we eat affects our energy levels. Until recently we were advised to eat a low-fat diet. As a result, anyone who wanted to lose weight started to eat anything that said 'low-fat'.

We have been doing that now for three decades, and how's it going? Are we trimmer, more healthy? No. We are more overweight, and the tsunami of diabetes is hitting our shores. Type 2 diabetes is a lifestyle disease. It is based on our lifestyle habits and what we eat.

The health industry and the food industry have encouraged us to "take personal responsibility" for our health. If we are overweight it is *our* fault. *We* need to watch what we eat, and exercise more.

I no longer blame anyone for being overweight after I was re-educated about our food. Our fast food industry is creating fake foods that are so addictive that people just go back for more like a cocaine addict goes back for his or her next fix.

Think about the man in the movie *Supersize Me*. He made a commitment to eat fast food for 30 days. The first few days he was vomiting after meals, like a teenager who drank too much. Then towards the end, his cholesterol increased and he gained 30 pounds. Most significantly, he felt depressed, tired, and irritable if he didn't go and eat another supersized fast food meal. What happened? He had become addicted to the junk food.

David Kessler MD, former head of the American Food and Drug Administration, wrote about this in *The End of Overeating*. In it he describes the science of how food is made into drugs by creating hyper-palatable foods that lead to chemical addictions. People are becoming addicted to junk food and we are getting bigger and sicker.

On the flip side people say, "No, you still have to take personal responsibility for being fat." Well then, what do we say about a three-year-old who is obese? What personal responsibility does that child need to exert? Obese children are fat because of the foods they are given. If children live in a food desert – predominant in poor neighbourhoods lacking fresh fruit and vegetable stores – then they are at more risk of obesity.

I have been addicted to French fries and hamburgers in the past, but I got some education under my belt and decided to take back my health. Now I want to lay a basic nutrition foundation which you too can build on.

So let's talk about your blood sugar levels. Research shows that low blood sugar levels are associated with lower overall blood flow to the brain, which means more bad decisions. Let's take a look at the graph below (Figure 1) to understand why we keep wanting to eat after consuming certain foods.

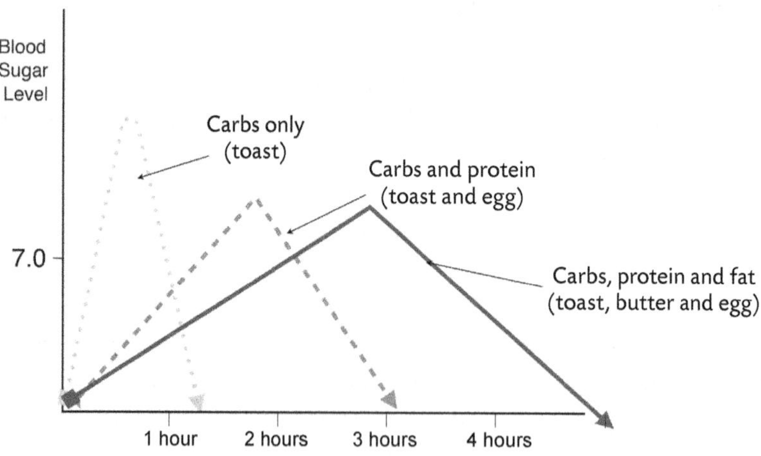

Figure 1: Blood Sugar Levels

Our blood sugar levels are affected by what we eat. Our body tells us when we are hungry based on our blood sugar levels. Our body's goal is to keep our blood sugars at a certain level. If they fall too low, then a message is sent to eat food.

Eating Carbohydrates

When we eat a carbohydrate, for instance a piece of toast, our blood sugar spikes. Within 60–90 minutes our blood sugar has fallen and we need to eat again. That's why when our kids are drinking an energy drink, which has about 7–13 teaspoons of sugar per drink, and a piece of toast or cereal for breakfast, they will be looking for food in 60–90 minutes. They have just consumed carbohydrates.

I am not saying not to eat carbs. Carbohydrates are very important for our wellbeing. But the *right* carbohydrates are more important.

Another point to keep in mind is this. When we eat carbs, the hormone *insulin* is released from the pancreas. The carbohydrate spike stimulates insulin, which has one major purpose: to store excess sugar as fat. Insulin will store fat anywhere, but it particularly loves to store belly fat.

Eating Carbohydrate + Protein

Now we add a protein such as egg with our toast. This stops us being hungry for at least 2.5–3 hours. As you can see in Figure 1, there is less of a spike in our blood sugar level, which results in less insulin release. The smaller the insulin spike, the less belly fat.

Eating Carbohydrate + Protein + Fat

Now we add some butter to our toast. Our blood sugar levels extend further and do not start dropping until 3.5–4 hours. So we won't start looking for more food to eat to get our blood sugar levels up.

Take a look at the insulin level when you eat a carb + protein + fat. Here we see less of an insulin spike, therefore less insulin is released, resulting in less belly fat! Isn't the body amazing!

In summary, the reason we see so much obesity has a lot to do with the fact that people are eating only carbohydrates. After about an hour they are hungry again because their blood sugars are going down and their bodies are screaming, "Find me more food!" We are very obedient and go to the fastest form of food for the fastest form of energy. Then insulin spikes, and there you have it … more belly fat.

What are Carbohydrates, Proteins and Fats?

Carbohydrates

- Flour in bread, scones, biscuits, pastries and pasta
- Sugar in candy or lollies, honey, jam, etc
- Legumes: kidney beans, chickpeas, baked beans, black beans
- Potatoes, sweet potatoes, kumara, pumpkin, taro, parsnips
- Veggies and fruit as in corn, peas, bananas, watermelon, pineapple
- Beer, wine, spirits
- Fruit juice and energy drinks

Proteins

- Meat: pork, lamb, chicken, beef
- Fish: tuna, salmon, etc
- Eggs
- Dairy: yoghurt (plain), cheese, cottage cheese, cream cheese
- Tofu
- Nuts: peanuts, almonds, cashews, walnuts, macadamia
- Seeds: pumpkin, sesame, chia seeds

Fats

- Fat on meat
- Chicken skin
- Lard
- Butter
- Margarine
- Oil: coconut oil, olive oil, canola oil, sesame oil, etc
- Salad dressings
- Mayonnaise

Now you have the basics of what constitutes a carbohydrate, protein and fat. You need to have all three of these every 3–4 hours to keep your blood sugars stable. By doing so you won't have those sharp blood sugar spikes which spike your insulin and result in belly fat accumulation.

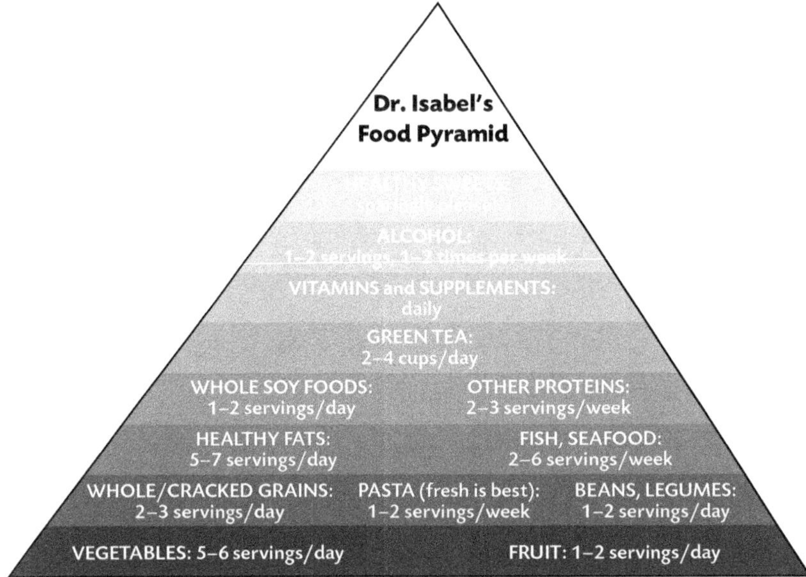

Figure 2: Dr. Isabel's Food Pyramid

People find the above diagram easy to use. Pay particular attention to the foundation of the pyramid. It consists of 5–6 servings of vegetables and 1–2 servings of fruit per day. *Every* day is the goal.

Taking back your health is much like remodelling your home. You can redecorate every room, but if there are cracks in the floors and walls from the foundation, your house will just keep sagging until eventually it collapses. If you get the foundation right, the rest will stand and endure. When storms come, the home will still be standing.

This is just like life. When the storms of life come, your health remodelling will enable you to endure and come out standing firm.

3. Why and How Our Bodies Store Fat

The reason our bodies store fat is to have a reserve of energy for the next famine. The problem is, there never is a famine – but your body doesn't know that. It is very obedient, and will do anything and everything to keep you alive. Whenever there's a surplus of food, it will get stored as fat for that day when there is no food.

Sugar in any form stimulates the release of insulin, a hormone that is stored in your pancreas. Insulin then causes an enzyme by the name of lipoprotein lipase (LPL) to store the excess sugar as fat.

Stress, on the other hand, stimulates the release of cortisol, which also stimulates LPL and results in the storage of fat.

What constitutes stress in your body? Anything that elevates your cortisol. Things like caffeine, sleep deprivation, too much exercise, work demands, family problems, financial difficulties, marriage conflict – just to name a few. Yes, stress can make you fat. The key is to recognise it and work to minimise it.

So in order to lose weight, the take-home message is that we need to decrease our sugar intake and our stress.

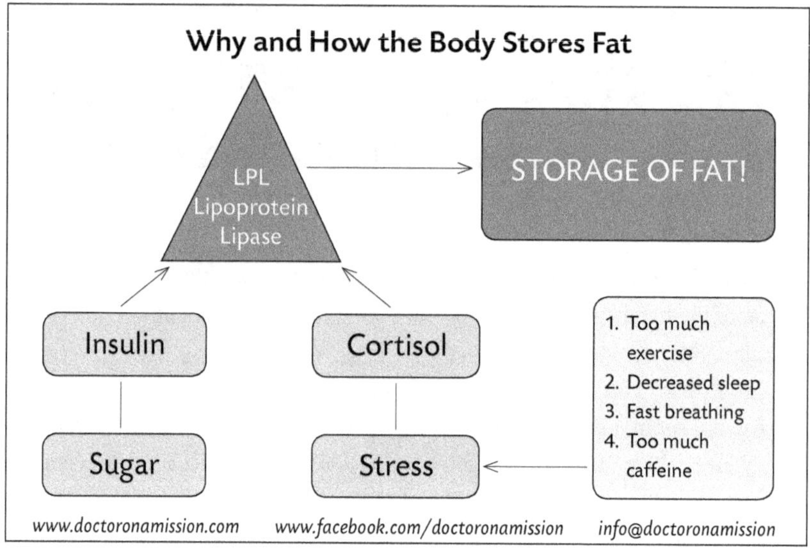

Fig 3: Why and how the body stores fat

The Cheating Rule

We have to have a time when we can splurge, like when we go out for a party or we are at a nice restaurant with beautiful breads, desserts, etc. For me it's usually on a Friday evening when I have been good all week with my food intake, then I let go. I splurge, and I do it without feeling guilty.

According to Dr. Heller at Mount Sinai Medical School in *The Great Physician* by Jordan Rubin, we can eat whatever we want if it is done within one hour. The rationale is this. They say that since your body has been used to low levels of sugar, less insulin is released, therefore less fat is stored – and more fat is used up for immediate energy. However at 75–90 minutes a second surge of insulin is released which results in fat storage.

Bottom line: If you are going to indulge, you have one hour to do it. After one hour, you will be packing it away as fat.

This does not mean that you can indulge every day for one hour. It means that if you need to go for it, you can do it once in a while without feeling like you blew it – but just do it within an hour. As your health coach I also encourage you to be good to your body, and not pig out on fast food or processed foods.

4. What Do I Eat, Doc?

What is GI?

Every day your body has to take more than 10,000 steps, think 40,000 thoughts, pump 36,000 litres of blood round your system to keep you alive for the next day. To do this it needs fuel, and our fuel – in the form of energy – comes from food.

Glucose is your body's preferred fuel source. It gets glucose from starches and sugars (carbohydrates) found in the food you eat every day. Glucose is made in the liver after your food has been digested in your stomach. The glucose is then sent wherever energy is needed in your body. This energy could be used for running or thinking, or it could be stored in muscles and fat for a later time.

The rate at which glucose goes into the bloodstream is called the 'glycemic index'.

- Low-glycemic index (low-GI) foods are converted slowly into glucose.
- Hi-glycemic index (high-GI) foods are converted quickly into glucose.

Insulin is very important in this whole process. I consider insulin to be the conductor of an orchestra made up of glucose particles.

When the glucose is released slowly (low-GI) there is no problem – the insulin has time to 'think' about where that glucose is needed most, and sends it there. But if high levels of glucose enter the bloodstream, the body 'panics'. It might need some of the glucose for fuel, but too much can be harmful. The body therefore releases more insulin, which quickly transfers the excess glucose to the fat stores where it can do no harm. As a result, we gain weight in the form of fat.

Weight gain isn't the only side effect of eating high-GI foods. If insulin levels are raised too often, then the cells that normally respond to glucose laugh at the insulin and say, "I'm not paying attention to you any more because you're always knocking on my door telling me to let the glucose in." Put another way, the cells become resistant to insulin's signals. This is called 'insulin resistance'.

Insulin resistance causes you to gain belly fat, raises your blood pressure, messes up your cholesterol, makes you infertile, kills your sex drive, makes you depressed, tired, demented, and even causes cancer.

When glucose is not allowed into the cells then a problem arises. The glucose remains in the bloodstream and causes damage – damage in the form of ageing and furring of the arteries. In addition, because the cells aren't getting enough fuel, causing you to feel tired, your body triggers the release of more and more insulin to try and fix up the problem. Over the years this triggers Type 2 diabetes.

The goal is to switch to eating low-GI foods, which will cause a gentle rise of glucose in your bloodstream. This will result in a balanced system and weight loss.

Below is a list of foods grouped into the traffic light system.

- **Low-GI foods** are considered Green Light: Eat as much as you want
- **Medium-GI foods** are considered Yellow Light: Eat in moderation
- **High-GI foods** are considered Red Light: Eat only as a treat
- **Extra High-GI foods** are considered Flashing Red Lights: Stay away!

GI FOOD LIST

Low-GI/Green Light: Eat large amounts

VEGETABLES: Broccoli, asparagus, spinach, chard, kale, cabbage, bok choy, carrots, eggplant, cauliflower, mushrooms, capsicums, lettuce, green beans, onions, leeks, types of seaweed, celery, sprouts, artichoke, courgettes/zucchini, cucumber, endive, fennel, garlic, leeks, rocket greens, watercress, radicchio, radish, tomato, spinach, boiled sweet potato/kumara.

WHOLE GRAINS: oat bran, rolled oats, pearl barley, quinoa, buckwheat.

LEGUMES/NUTS: Chickpeas, peanuts, walnuts, cashews, almonds, kidney beans, butter beans, navy beans, pinto beans, lentils, black beans, yellow spilt peas, soy beans.

FRUIT: Grapefruit, kiwi fruit, coconut, apples, avocado, all berries (like blueberries, strawberries, boysenberries, etc), plums, green grapes, cherries.

PROTEIN *(Please note that the following are certainly categorised as low-GI, however I caution you regarding the fat content):* Anchovies, bacon, beef, chicken, clams, cod, crab, duck, eggs, gammon, haddock, halibut, ham, kippers, lamb, liver, lobster, mackerel, monkfish, mussels, pilchards, plaice, pork, prawns, salmon, sardines, sea bass, skate, squid, sole, swordfish, trout, tuna, venison, veal.

Medium-GI/Yellow Light: Eat in moderation

VEGETABLES: Beets/beetroot.

WHOLE GRAINS: Brown rice, basmati rice, black rice, red rice, couscous.

FRUIT: Peaches, nectarines, mango, apricots, pears, papaya, figs, melons, red grapes.

High-GI/Red Light: Eat only as a treat

VEGETABLES: Baked potato, baked sweet potato/kumara, boiled potato, winter squash, peas, broad beans (fava), pumpkin, turnips, yams.

WHOLE GRAINS: Any rice that takes 10 minutes or less to cook, jasmine rice, sticky rice, millet.

FRUIT: Watermelon, dates, pineapple, bananas. *(Did you know that one banana has 4.25 teaspoons of sugar?)*

Extra High-GI/Flashing Red Light: Stay away!

Dried fruit and candy (lollies).

DRINKS AND GI

It's not only food that turns into glucose in your body. Drinks do too.
Below is a list of Low-GI to High-GI drinks.

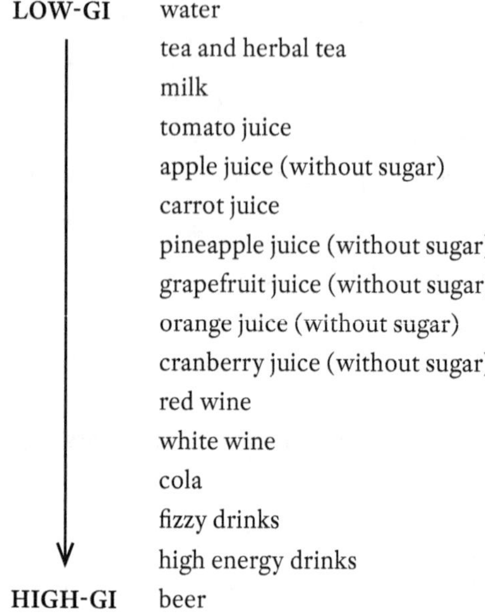

About alcoholic drinks

Alcoholic drinks in the form of spirits such as gin, vodka and whiskey are also best avoided. While they have very little effect on insulin – they are technically low-GI – they increase our appetite, resulting in overeating. In addition, high consumption of spirits is linked to other health problems.

Red wine is a better choice than spirits. Although it has a medium-GI value, it contains antioxidants, which are good for your heart.

About fats

We also need to focus on which fats are safe to consume. There is a lot of confusion out there regarding which fats are ok to eat and which are ok to cook with. Below is a list for your kitchen.

FOOD SOURCES OF GOOD AND BAD FATS

GOOD Essential Fats

OMEGA-3: Flax, soybean, walnuts, organic expeller-pressed canola oil, dark green leafy veggies, cold water fish (cod, salmon, sardines, anchovies, tuna), pumpkin.

OMEGA-6: Cold-pressed flax and sunflower oil, cold-pressed high oleic safflower oil, walnuts, grapeseed oil, sesame oil and tahini.

GOOD Monounsaturated Fats

Extra-virgin cold-pressed olive oil, sesame oil, brazil nuts, hazelnuts and filberts, avocado, peanuts and peanut butter (non-hydrogenated and no added sugar), cashews, almonds and almond butter, macadamia nuts, walnuts, pine nuts, soybean oil, organic expeller-pressed canola oil.

GOOD Saturated Fats

Ghee (clarified butter), poultry (chicken and turkey), coconut oil, butter.

BAD Trans Fats

Trans fats cause free radicals to be formed, causing damage to and ageing of your body.

Margarine, hydrogenated peanut butter, chocolate candy, pastries and doughnuts, commercially packaged cookies, crackers, and chips, shortening, any foods fried in shortening-type oils (deep-fried), corn, sunflower and canola oils that are not cold-pressed (they contain hydrogenated or partially hydrogenated oils).

BAD Saturated and Processed Fats

Shortening, all partially hydrogenated oils, rancid oils (smelling bad, exposed to oxygen) – *all oils left exposed to oxygen can go rancid, which may be toxic to human tissue,* poultry skin, cheese, red meats (beef, pork, lamb), high temperature deep-fried foods, all hydrogenated oils.

Best Oils to Cook with at High Temperature

Coconut oil, expeller or cold-pressed sesame oil, expeller or cold-pressed sunflower oil.

As you can see, butter is better than margarine. Margarine is not a whole food, rather it is a trans fat which causes the formation of free radicals in your body, which do all kinds of damage. Free radical formation, in particular, causes your body to age in fast-forward motion. If you put a block of margarine and butter out for the ants, they eat the butter and don't touch the margarine. So stay away from margarine and use butter.

"But what about my cholesterol, Doc?" Great question. There is recent research to indicate that we shouldn't be worried about our cholesterol as much as the things that cause inflammation (I will address inflammation in the next section). Half of all heart attack victims have normal cholesterol levels. So high cholesterol levels are *not* the cause of all the heart disease in the world.

Five Messages to Guide You to Health

1. Raw is best

Try your hardest to eat foods in their natural state. Consider how old the food you are buying is. Typically it has taken at least one week to get to you, so its nutritional value has already depleted by 40–50%. If you cook it, then again important enzymes and nutrients will be destroyed.

If steaming food a little is the best way to start your family on this journey, then I encourage that. In our family we have a motto to reach the goal: "Whatever it takes". However, the final goal is to eat foods in their freshest form, straight from the farmer's field. If you can eat organic, great! If not, then you can do the following to clean your fruits and veggies:

One part white vinegar to ten parts water.
Let sit for few minutes, then wash off.

This is the closest we can get to taking the pesticides off our food.

2. Eat foods without labels or that don't come in a box, can or package

If they do have labels then you need to make sure to read the labels very carefully. Ideally you want less than 5 ingredients.

3. Stay away from the following ingredients:

- Foods with **preservatives, additives, colouring** or **dyes.** Anything you can't pronounce or recognise is a big no-no.
- All foods containing **high fructose corn syrup.** Other disguised names for this are **corn syrup** or **sugar of maize** ('maize' is Spanish for corn). This is an industrial food product which is not natural, whole, real or fresh, and it lacks fibre or any nutritional value. In some cases mercury is a by-product. Who needs it? If you want to avoid obesity, stay far away from it.
- All **white rice** and **white flour.** White rice and white flour stimulate insulin release, and insulin's main purpose is to store fat for a future famine. It loves to store it where it can access it quickly: around the belly, upper arms, and the back (lovingly called *verandas*).
- **Sugar** in the form of honey, agave, maple syrup, cane sugar or molasses. Sugar in any form also causes a rise in insulin, which causes belly fat accumulation.
- Anything **hydrogenated.** This chemical process is just a way to add hydrogen atoms to fats so they survive longer on the shelf. It has been known to cause heart disease and cancer. Most European countries and even New York City have banned these fats, and I encourage you to do the same, for the sake of your health.
- Fried foods and processed oils such as corn, peanut and canola. These fats are toxic when heated and full of free radicals – which can actually change good DNA into damaged DNA. They have no nutritional value, so why even pour them into your tank?
- **Artificial sweeteners** such as:
  - Saccharin (sweet and low)
  - Anything that ends in 'ol' like xylitol, sorbitol, mannitol, lactitol, and mailtol
  - Acesulfame-k, known as *Ace-K, Sunette, Sweet and Safe* (not!) and *Sweet One.* These all slow down your metabolism, make you hungry and make you fat. In one study using two groups, one was given a diet drink and the other a non-diet drink every day. At the end of the year, those who had the diet drink gained the most weight.

5. What's all this talk about 'inflammation'?

As a medical doctor, I have been trained that a low fat and low cholesterol diet is the best prevention against heart disease, heart attacks, high blood pressure and obesity. After a patient was tested and found to have high cholesterol levels we then put them on a statin, which lowers the cholesterol levels, and we started the patient on a low fat diet. Put so eloquently by Dr. Dwight Lundell, a heart surgeon in USA, "To deviate from this was considered heresy and could quite possibly result in malpractice."

But the low fat, low cholesterol plan is not working. Half of all those who have heart attacks have normal cholesterol levels. Today people are sicker than ever before, and now we know that it's all preventable.

What do we know about the childhood problem? Childhood obesity has tripled in the thirty years from 1980 to 2010. One in three children born today will have Type 2 diabetes in their lifetime. Childhood obesity will have more impact on how long this generation will live than all childhood cancers. Childhood diabetes is a global problem. 60% of the world's Type 2 diabetics will be from Asia because it's the world's largest region.

Fortunately there have been new studies which show us that we had the low fat, low cholesterol plan *all wrong*. Inflammation is the cause.

A mental picture of inflammation

Imagine a stiff brush rubbing on skin over a short period of time. The skin breaks down and starts to bleed. This causes the body's repair system to come in and start repairing the injured area. The area becomes red, hot and swollen for a short period of time, and then heals up. This is the normal way our body repairs any injured site.

Now let's imagine that over a long period of time the brush is rubbing the inside of a blood vessel leading to your heart. What happens is the area becomes sticky, and when cholesterol comes floating by it hooks onto the sticky area on the blood vessel. Over time more and more cholesterol hooks on, eventually blocking the blood vessel leading to the heart. Then you get a heart attack. A heart attack is nothing more than a lack of blood supply to the heart muscle.

The main point here is this: The cholesterol is not the problem, the stiff brush is. It's the stiff brush that created the whole problem. We need cholesterol for everyday life to make every living cell in our body. If I could take you and me right now into a living cell in your body, we would see that cholesterol makes the walls of that cell's 'house'. If we didn't have cholesterol, we couldn't be alive.

What are the 'stiff brushes' that are causing all this havoc in our body? Or, put another way, what are the creators of inflammation?

1. **SUGAR.** Sugar is found in almost everything we eat. It is in bread, fast food with high fructose corn syrup, energy drinks, colas, pasta, and on and on and on. We know that sugar stimulates insulin, which does one of two things:
   - It stores sugar into cells, and when that is all done …
   - it stores sugar as fat. If you are insulin-resistant than the sugar can't get into the cells and stays in the bloodstream.

   Sugar in the bloodstream is dangerous because it starts scratching the inside of the blood vessel, just like the stiff brush. It makes it sticky and ready for cholesterol to hook on and cause problems.
   Sugar also wipes out your immune system for up to 2–4 hours after eating it. Your immune system is your army inside you, attacking viruses and bacteria that come into your body. You don't want your army asleep when it's invaded by viruses and bacteria.

2. **HIGH-FAT FOODS.** Especially foods high in trans fats, saturated fats and processed fats – like the deep fried foods we see and eat in fast food restaurants and takeaway fish and chip stores.

3. **FOOD ALLERGENS.** People who are allergic to certain foods form immune complexes which lead to inflammation. Common food allergens include gluten, soy, dairy, peanut, eggs and artificial sweeteners, to name a few.

4. **INSUFFICIENT FIBRE.** Think of fibre as a broom in your gut sweeping out toxins that cause inflammation.

5. **INSUFFICIENT PHYTONUTRIENTS.** *Phyto* means plant. Phytonutrients are plant nutrients that are beneficial to you. Phytonutrients found in fruits, vegetables, nuts and seeds act to quench inflammation.

6. **INSUFFICIENT EXERCISE.** Fat tissue helps to hide the contributors to inflammation. Exercising muscle reduces inflammation and improves insulin's delivery of glucose to cells.

7. **VITAMIN D3 DEFICIENCY.** This important vitamin has been found to be a prime player in the prevention of inflammation. More on this in detail in Chapter 7.

8. **EMOTIONAL STRESS.** Emotional stress and toxic relationships promote inflammation, slow down wound healing and suppress your immune system.

The bottom line is that it's not the fat or cholesterol in our diets that is causing heart disease, high blood pressure, Type 2 diabetes, strokes, obesity, or Alzheimer's disease. The real cause is inflammation. People have been on a low fat, low cholesterol diet for six decades, and it just isn't working.

So, what do we do? Only eat foods that our great great grandmothers would recognise.

CHAPTER TWO

Healthy Shopping

1. What to Have in Your Kitchen

It's time to get your kitchen ready for your success. I suggest getting rid of all the bad stuff and investing in all the good stuff for your health and future. You're worth it.

Utensils

Blender, non-aluminium cooking pans, wooden cutting board, sharp knives, measuring spoons.

Spices *(make sure these don't have any preservatives or sugar added to them)*

Salt, pepper, oregano, basil, paprika, cumin, chilli powder, curry powder, rosemary, cinnamon, turmeric.

Oils/Sauces to have on hand

Extra virgin olive oil cold pressed, organic soy or tamari sauce (wheat free), coconut oil, sesame oil cold pressed, sunflower oil cold pressed, balsamic vinegar, butter.

Pantry

Garlic cloves, sweet potatoes/kumara, red and white onions, ginger root

Tea

Organic green tea, peppermint tea, ginger tea.

Nuts *(raw, not roasted, as roasting reduces nutritional value)*

Almonds, walnuts, brazil nuts, peanuts (if not allergic), pine nuts, chia seeds, sesame seeds, sunflower seeds, pumpkin seeds, macadamia nuts, oconut (shredded, without sugar), pecans.

Grains

Brown rice, red rice, black rice, quinoa, oats.

Legumes/Beans *(canned is ok)*

Chickpeas, kidney beans, black beans, butter beans, lentils, navy beans, pinto beans, yellow split beans, soy beans.

Miscellaneous

Coconut milk (without sugar), almond milk (without sugar), hemp milk, oat milk, tahini (ground sesame), organic almond butter, organic peanut butter, anchovy, capers, mustard, mayonnaise (without sugar), tomato sauce.

Breakfast Cereal

Have a rolled oat cereal without sugar on hand for kids.

Refrigerator

Grapefruit, kiwifruit, strawberries, blueberries, boysenberries, grapes, apples, cherries, peaches, nectarines, mangoes, apricots, pears, papaya, melon, broccoli, asparagus, spinach, chard, kale, cabbage, bok choy, carrots, eggplant, cauliflower, mushrooms, red pepper/capsicums, lettuce, green beans, leeks, celery, sprouts, artichoke, courgettes/zucchini, cucumber, endive, fennel, rocket greens, watercress, radicchio, radish, beets/beetroot.

Protein

Eggs, chicken breasts, tofu, salmon, tuna, clams, mussels, fish, grass-fed beef, lamb, duck.

2. Places Where Sugar Hides

When I met up with one of my clients for health coaching, I asked her to remove sugar from her life. She said to me so innocently, "Oh, I never add sugar to anything." I looked at her lovingly and said, "You don't have to, the food industry does it for you!"

You almost need a PhD to go shopping nowadays, what with sugar's multitude of aliases. Below is a list for you to have while shopping. Even my 13-year-old patients carry it with them, and are so excited to be on the hunt for sugar in their food. They know that sugar stimulates insulin release, which causes more belly fat to be stored.

Here's the list of sugar's many hiding places:

- Agave syrup or Agave sugar *(Yes, agave has a low GI, however what it does is far worse than raise insulin levels. It increases your triglyceride levels, triggering inflammation and damaging your liver.)*
- Barley malt
- Beet sugar
- Brown sugar
- Buttered syrup
- Cane juice crystals
- Cane sugar
- Caramel
- Corn syrup
- Corn syrup solids
- Confectioner's sugar
- Carob syrup
- Castor sugar
- Date sugar
- Demerara sugar
- Dextran
- Dextrose
- Diastatic malt
- Diatese
- Dried fruit (high glucose and concentrated sugar)
- Ethyl maltol

- Fructose
- Fruit juice
- Fruit juice concentrate
- Galactose
- Glucose
- Glucose solids
- Golden sugar
- Golden syrup
- Grape sugar
- High fructose corn syrup (HFCS)
- Sugar of maize
- Honey
- Icing sugar
- Invert sugar
- Lactose
- Maltodextrin
- Maltose
- Malt syrup
- Maple syrup
- Molasses
- Muscovado sugar
- Panocha
- Raw sugar
- Refiner's syrup
- Rice syrup
- Sorbitol
- Sorghum syrup
- Sucrose
- Sugar
- Treacle
- Turbinado sugar
- Xylitol
- Yellow sugar
- Anything ending in '–ose' is a sugar

Now the question arises: "What can I use as a sweetener?" I always recommend *stevia*. Stevia, a plant from the sunflower family, is 300 times sweeter than sugar. It is low-GI and if you need something as a sweetener, then stevia is your best option. This is what we use in our family. I prefer the drops as I can control the sweetness more readily.

3. What Foods to Buy

Making the decision to take better care of yourself through healthy eating is the first step. I always like to think of my body as a car: if I pour concrete into the gasoline tank, I won't get very far. However, when I 'fill her up' with high octane, I will get far. The same philosophy applies to our bodies.

I was born in 1959, and I am just about to turn 53 years young. My family is from Cuba, and in Cuba the cars last a long time. If I were to consider myself like a 1959 Ford Fairlane which I had to keep running for a long time, I would take really good care of myself.

I haven't always filled my tank with high octane. I wasn't even in the right headspace to do that, especially during my medical education. Breakfast for me was dessert – a strong cup of coffee and a muffin. We know that after that nutritious breakfast my blood sugars were falling again within 1.5 hours. Nothing a handful of candy and another cup of coffee couldn't handle, which would hold me over for another 1.5 hours.

Rollercoaster blood sugars not only feel bad, they just play havoc with your emotions. Think about our kids in school who have had dessert for breakfast. From my window I used to see kids going to school with bags of chips and an energy drink. Not only would I feel sorry for the kids, but also for the poor teachers. It's impossible for the kids to concentrate. Hence the need to create your new health strategy, and reposition yourself for better health.

Repositioning yourself and your family is a little tricky. It's much like making an ocean liner do a 180-degree turn – not a quick manoeuvre. I remember when I foolishly announced to my teenage daughters that I wasn't going to buy any more sugar. I was crucified! It was like taking away a drug from the drug addict – and in a way I was.

Like Robert Kiyosaki says, "You either win or you learn!" I learned that I shouldn't have announced to the Hunsinger Home my new commitment of 'no sugar' . . . I should just have implemented it quietly. Allow yourself time for the reposition. Once completed, you will be on the right track.

Buying Organic

I am completely amazed at how expensive organic food can be at times. I would purposely avoid going into the organic shops because I thought it was only for the rich who could afford to waste their money on expensive foods. Remember, I did my pre-med degree in Boulder, Colorado.

After reading and researching, however, I have learned so much more about organic food. The organic farmer is held to a set of stringent rules, and is not subsidised by the government. Organic farms produce a higher quality of food without added chemicals or genetic modification. Quite honestly, I cannot un-learn what I have learned, and I would be lying to you if I coached you otherwise: When possible, I would encourage you to buy organic. You are worth the investment.

If it's difficult to purchase organic greens and vegetables in your area, as it is with us, then you can clean your purchases with one part white vinegar and ten parts water. Just swish around for a few minutes then rinse in water. That process will help remove most of the pesticides. Remember, we do whatever we have to in order to achieve the goal. Step by step.

CHAPTER THREE

Healthy Cooking with Chef Michael

Yummy food that your body and your family will love

1. Kitchen Essentials and Time-Saving Tips

Here is a list of my kitchen essentials:

- Sharp set of knives
- Cutting board (preferably two; one for protein, one for all the rest)
- Food processor
- Drink blender
- Utensils: whisk, spoon, spatula, etc.
- Fresh herbs and spices, including sea salt and black pepper
- Fresh garlic and ginger
- Set of bowls for mixing
- Set of measuring cups and spoons
- Extra virgin olive oil (cold pressed) for non-cooking recipes
- Sesame oil and coconut oil for cooking

Timesaving Tips for a Busy Life

It seems that with all our wonderful gadgets and modern conveniences, life should be simpler and full of free time. I've noticed, however, that most people today live busier lives than they did 20 years ago. One pleasure we often miss out on today is eating Healthy Real Food Meals. I'm not going to try and analyse why this is happening (though I do have an opinion). Let's look at some techniques that will help you organise your time in the kitchen, so hopefully you can sit, relax, and enjoy Real 100% Food.

- Prepare a mixed raw vegetable platter on Sunday and Thursday with a dipping sauce or hummus (prep time about one hour). This will allow the family to have a healthy snack ready at all times to be eaten at home or taken to school or work: tomato quarters, carrot and celery sticks, broccoli and cauliflower lightly steamed and cooled, capsicum strips (bell pepper), zucchini strips (courgette), etc.
- Soups, sauces, and salads – I like to prepare these items in larger quantities to last a few days. Soups and sauces can be frozen and used another time. Salads are great for two days without the lettuce (which will wilt).
- Prepare a few extra portions when making a main dish, and freeze some. Generally, if I'm going to take the time to cook and get into the kitchen, then I want to make my time count. It doesn't take more time to prepare extra when I already have the ingredients and food cooking. Making two litres of soup takes pretty much the same time as making one litre of soup.

2. Breakfast, Your Day's Important Start

Breakfast is the most important meal of the day – it jumpstarts your metabolism and gets bodily functions on the correct path. Start your day with a healthy breakfast within one hour of awakening, and you will have an energised, healthy, tuned-in day. Here are some recommended ways to start your day.

— PROTEIN SHAKE —

We recommend using a dairy-free or rice/pea protein if you are overweight. We know from research that rice/pea protein helps burn body fat, and is hypoallergenic.

Healthy Starter

1–2 scoops protein powder
mixed fruit berries, 2 cups
tahini paste, 1 Tbs.
chia seeds, 2 Tbs. (high in omega-3 fatty acids and fibre)
pinch of cinnamon
non-dairy milk, 2 cups (almond, rice, coconut, hemp – all without sugar)
water or ice cubes, 2 cups

Blend all in drink mixer and enjoy. Makes 2–3 servings.

Mocha-Blueberry

1–2 scoops of protein powder
1 cup of blueberries
1 cup organic decaf plunger or espresso coffee
pinch of cinnamon
2 Tbs. chia seeds
2 cups non-dairy milk
2 cups water or ice

Blend all to make 2–3 servings.

Strawberry-Coconut Desire

Use the healthy starter recipe with these changes:
- *only strawberries for fruit*
- *use coconut milk*
- *add 2 Tbs. of coconut flakes*

Blend all to make 2–3 servings.

— VEGETABLE FRITTATA (no crust quiche) —

This can be made the day before and reheated.

10 eggs whisked in bowl
2 cups diced vegetables
2 garlic cloves chopped
2 Tbs. fresh chopped parsley
2 Tbs. fresh chopped basil
1 Tbs. dry dill leaf
salt and pepper to taste

Sauté veggies for 3 minutes with garlic and herbs. When done, combine veggie and egg mixture in a lightly buttered baking pan. Bake in oven at 150°C (325°F) for 25–35 min (nice golden brown).

SUGGESTED FLAVOURS: bacon or ham, grated cheese, salmon pieces, mushrooms, capsicum, onion, courgettes, tomato.

— PLAIN GREEK YOGHURT —

Another great option for breakfast is plain Greek yoghurt. Greek yoghurt has more protein than regular yoghurt, and by adding a few ingredients you can have a protein-filled meal. Add flaxseed or chia seeds for the omega-3s, fresh berries, organic muesli mix, and two drops of stevia for sweetness.

— QUICK AND EASY —

If you want to keep it simple, have two eggs poached on 1 piece of gluten-free buttered toast. That will do you for the morning.

3. Juice Recipes for Fast/Cleanse

In 2012 Michael and I, along with some friends from around the world, did a 10-day juice fast. Yes, no chewing of food for 10 days; yes, just real 100% juice. Before you turn off, thinking "that's crazy!", please understand that the health reasons for a juice fast are many, and your body will truly love what it does for your organs. We have decided to keep our Tuesdays as Juice Fast Day, as we love the cleansing and energising effect we get during this process. Here are some recipes we have used for our juice fast. I hope you enjoy them if you choose to 'juice'.

Quick Tips

- When the recipe calls for fruit, please make fruit a maximum 20% of your blend.
- Using wheatgrass gives a high octane of nutrients to any juice.
- Adding cracked black pepper and sea salt adds to the flavour.

— THE KIWIANA —

Blend of beetroot (red beets), kale, red radishes, carrots, and apples.

— MORNING ZINGER —

Apples, carrots, celery, orange, fresh ginger.

— THE THIRST QUENCHER —

Green apple, kale or spinach, cucumber, celery, lime.

— THE ITALIAN —

Tomatoes, capsicum (bell pepper), spinach or kale, celery, garlic clove, fresh basil, fresh parsley.

— THE LATIN FIRE —

Tomatoes, cucumber, spinach or kale, celery, carrots, fresh chilli peppers, garlic clove, pinch of cumin seed, pinch of smoked paprika.

4. Soups, Sauces, Dips

Let's have fun with soups, sauces, and dips. This is one of my favorite areas of food, because we can experiment with so many flavours. All of the recipes can be made in bulk, so you can freeze them for future use. I will add some flavour suggestions to each recipe, however please feel free to try new tastes on your own.

— SAUCES & DIPS —

Traditional Hummus

This is one of my favourite foods because it has the right combination of protein, carbs and good fats. It can be used as a spread for sandwiches, or as a dip for veggies and crackers.

2 cups cooked or canned chickpeas (garbanzo beans)
½ cup liquid from chickpeas
Juice of 1 lemon
1 clove garlic
2 Tbs. chopped parsley
2 Tbs. extra virgin olive oil
2 Tbs. tahini
Salt and pepper to taste

Purée all ingredients in food processor.

SUGGESTED FLAVOURS *(you can use one or more):* Sundried tomatoes, roasted red capsicum, diced beetroot, rocket leaves, olives, extra garlic clove.

Basic Aioli

4 egg yolks
2 cups extra virgin olive oil
1 garlic clove
juice of 1 lemon
salt and pepper to taste

Purée all ingredients except oil in food processor, then slowly add oil to purée until desired thickness. Listen to the machine start to work harder as the aioli thickens, and turn off the machine once you reach the desired thickness.

SUGGESTED FLAVOURS: Capsicum or chillies, olives, fresh basil or parsley, extra garlic clove, fresh coriander, fresh lime juice.

Traditional Pasta/Pizza sauce

1 diced onion
4 garlic cloves
about 12 fresh basil leaves chopped
small bunch fresh parsley chopped
6 large diced tomatoes or 2 cans of chopped tomatoes
salt and pepper to taste

Sauté all ingredients except tomatoes for 3–5 minutes, add tomatoes, turn down low, and simmer for 30 minutes. Serves 8.

SUGGESTED FLAVOURS: Fresh oregano, fresh thyme, different types of tomatoes, add some chopped courgette (zucchini), or diced carrots and capsicum (bell peppers).

– SOUPS –

Soup is another one of my favourites. I will provide a basic recipe to start with, and then you can have fun from there. Soup is an inexpensive way to feed the family healthily at any time of the year. Just use the products that are in season.

Quick/Simple Vegetable Soup

About a litre or medium bowl of coarsely chopped vegetables
a litre of vegetable stock
herbs and spices to taste

Sauté vegetables, herbs, and spices in large pot for about 5 minutes. Add stock and simmer for 30 minutes. Purée in drink blender or with hand-held food blender to desired thickness. Season to taste.

HOT TIP: Add kumara (yams) or cauliflower to vegetable mix, as they are slightly starchy and will thicken the soup naturally. Have fun and use many types and flavours of vegetables and fresh herbs.

Asian Tom Yum Soup

Ingredients for 2 litres:
2 cups thinly sliced or diced chicken
1–2 chopped hot chilli (depending on your preferred heat level)
julienne of 1 red and 1 green capsicum
1 carrot diced or Asian cut
2 sticks celery Asian cut or diced
1 cup sliced shitake mushrooms
¼ cup green peas
¼ cup sliced green onions
1 litre chicken stock
2 cans coconut cream
4 Tbs. fresh grated ginger
6 cloves garlic
salt and pepper to taste

Sauté chicken, vegetables and spices for 5 minutes, add stock, continue to simmer soup for 15 minutes, then add coconut cream and lime juice, season to taste, simmer for 15–30 minutes more. You can take 25% of soup and blend in drink blender. Add the mix back into the soup to thicken, and finish.

5. Lunch/Dinner

Yes, I have purposely put lunch and dinner sections together. The western diet seems to pack in most of our food intake at the end of our waking day. This isn't the healthy way to distribute our daily calorie intake. And many people consume more just before going to bed. This is like throwing a huge log on a fire with low embers. You lose the fire and just get smoke.

So we store fat at the end of the day because we aren't moving much (usually we're sitting watching TV). Unless you are doing a tango competition from 9pm–midnight, you won't be burning much energy after 8pm. We should have about 70% of our daily calorie intake by the time we have our dinner. So let's look at the lunch/dinner recipes as interchangeable.

— STIR-FRY CHICKEN —

Marinated chicken pieces (marinate in coriander, lime, garlic,
coconut cream or coconut milk, fresh ginger, tamari or soy sauce)
Mixture of sliced and diced veggies
Brown, long grain, red or black rice

Stir-fry chicken in hot pan using coconut, sesame, or sunflower oil for 2–3 minutes, then add mixture of raw veggies. Stir-fry hot for about 5 minutes (try not to overcook the mix). Serve with cooked rice.

SUGGESTED FLAVOURS: celery, carrot, capsicum, green beans, broccoli, mushrooms, courgette, leeks, red onion, chilli peppers. Have fun with your veggie mix by using different types of cuts.

— GREEK SALAD —

1 red onion, 1 red capsicum, 1 green capsicum, 2 tomatoes, 1 cucumber
(all coarsely chopped)
handful of pitted green and black olives
50 grams of feta cheese

For salad dressing:
juice of 1 lemon
1 crushed garlic clove
1 Tbs. oregano
1 Tbs. chopped parsley

¼ cup extra virgin olive oil
cracked black pepper and sea salt to taste

In small mixing bowl, mix all salad dressing ingredients except oil. Then using a whisk, slowly blend in olive oil. In large salad bowl mix vegetables, herbs, spices and olives. Pour salad dressing over vegetable mix to desired wetness.

SUGGESTED SERVING: Place cos (romaine) lettuce leaves around edge of serving platter, place salad mix in middle, and top with crumbled feta cheese and chopped parsley leaves.

– QUINOA SALAD WITH AVOCADO AND BLACK BEANS –

1 cup quinoa
1½ cups water
1 chopped scallion (green onion)
½ diced red capsicum (bell pepper)
1 sliced tomato
1 sliced avocado
1 cup black beans (cooked)
2 limes
fresh coriander/cilantro
olive oil to taste
fresh rocket or spinach greens

Cook quinoa in lightly simmering water (salt and pepper to taste) for 5 minutes. Turn off heat and allow to sit covered for about 10–12 more minutes until water is absorbed. Some veggie stock or some butter in water for flavour is nice.

When quinoa is cool, combine with juice of 1 lime, red capsicum, scallion, 2 Tbs. olive oil, 1 Tbs. chopped coriander, pinch of dried cumin. Toss all ingredients in bowl.

TO SERVE: On serving tray place greens around edge, then alternate tomato and avocado slices to form colourful pattern. Place quinoa mixture in middle of platter, sprinkle black beans around edges, and garnish with sprinkle of chopped coriander and lime wedges. Drizzle some olive oil on greens and tomato/avocado pattern.

— COLESLAW —

½ head green cabbage shredded
¼ head red cabbage shredded
2 carrots shredded
1 red onion diced small
1 green capsicum diced small
½ cup basic aioli
juice of 1 lemon
fresh dill, parsley, salt, pepper to taste

Combine all ingredients in mixing bowl, and serve as side dish with main course. Makes enough for about 10 servings.

— BAKED FRESH SALMON FILLET —

The salmon can be eaten warm after baking, or cooled and eaten for salads, or with eggs for breakfast. Great protein dish full of Omega 3 fatty acids. I like to cook a large piece to have for meals over a day or two.

whole boneless salmon side, skin on
1 lemon
fresh or dry dill weed
smoked paprika

Lightly grease baking pan with sesame or coconut oil. Place salmon fillet on pan, spread spices, herbs, salt and pepper and juice of lemon over salmon. Bake in oven @ 150°C for about 15–20 minutes. The meat will be a lovely pink colour when finished. When cooled, the meat will come off the skin easily if desired.

— FISH AND CHIPS —

Yes, I know, how can that be healthy? Well, here is an alternative that is tasty, and remains nutritious.

4 pieces firm white flesh fish of your choice
3 golden kumara (yams) cut in wedges
gluten-free flour
gluten-free breadcrumbs
2 eggs for egg-wash
sesame or coconut oil

Dredge fish in flour, then into egg-wash (mixture of eggs and water), then into breadcrumbs. Place on plate and chill for 1 hour to set.

Cut kumara into wedges, about ⅛ the size. Toss them in a mix of paprika, garlic, chilli powder, salt and pepper, and 1 Tbs. sesame oil.

Bake kumara in 180°C oven for about 20 minutes.

Fry the fish fillets in sesame or coconut oil for 5 minutes, until golden brown.

Serve with aioli, or a wasabi mayo, and of course ketchup if you like.

— CHICKEN CAESAR SALAD —

This classic salad can be a main meal for lunch or dinner. You might also omit the chicken, and use as a side salad for the main meal. You could substitute salmon for chicken for a twist.

2 cups of diced or julienned chicken meat
2 pieces of gluten-free bread
fresh parmesan cheese
4 whole eggs
caesar-style aioli
1 head cos lettuce (romaine)

Wash, clean, and chop lettuce coarsely. Drain off excess water and set aside.

For the Caesar dressing use basic aioli recipe with addition of anchovy fillets, 1 extra garlic clove and some parmesan cheese.

Cut the bread into cubes and toss with enough melted butter to lightly moisten. Sauté in pan until nice golden brown for croutons. Cook the chicken meat and set aside. Poach the eggs and set aside.

TO SERVE: Toss lettuce leaves, chicken and croutons in mixing bowl with enough aioli to flavour them. Place mix on platter, place 1 poached egg on top per serving, and sprinkle grated parmesan over top. Serves 4 side salads or 2 main meals.

CHAPTER FOUR

Why Winners Win
The Mental Game of Winning Health

1. Attitude

> *The problem is not the problem. The problem is your attitude*
> *about the problem. Do you understand?*
> – Captain Jack Sparrow

Why do some people win and some people lose? I believe it all has to do with a person's attitude.

Here is a true-life example that I just experienced the other day while Michael and I were out on a walk. It was a beautiful warm sunny spring Saturday afternoon. I was in the middle of writing this book and Michael had a lot of projects on the go.

Michael is a peaceful, pleasant, easy-going and adaptable person. He's also fun, outgoing and optimistic. Nothing much rocks his boat. I'm also fun, outgoing and optimistic, but my stronger personality trait of being goal-oriented and bossy has a tendency to take over. And so it did on this walk.

In the middle of the walk I said, "OK, when we get back, we're going to buckle down and get to work." Michael smiled and said, "I prefer to say, I'm going to enjoy the day."

I was thinking about getting serious and buckling down and getting some work done. Someone once said that writing books is like having homework the rest of your life, and I can truly relate to this. And so, this attitude brought on a surge of anxiety in my heart.

Michael, on the other hand, still wanted to reach his goal of getting work done, but it was through enjoyment of the journey. I thank God for bringing a man into my life who brings peace and helps me think about what I'm thinking about.

The bottom line is that our attitude is the mental gymnastics we play. It is our thought life turned inside out. How you think will determine how you live your life – either enjoying the journey, or dreading it. Most people's minds are like a wild untamed animal. You just have to learn to tame your mind. You have to crave and pursue the taming of your mind. That is work, because it is an everyday event. Trust me, I constantly have to think about what I'm thinking. If my mind is not on the right track to reach my goal, then I have to change what I'm saying to myself.

We have control of two things in this world: our thoughts and our attitude. Those two determine where we go and where we end up.

I am always amazed and excited when I meet or read of someone who had terrible experiences, but decided to take control of their thoughts and attitude and become an overcomer.

Chris Gardner is a perfect example. He is portrayed in the movie *The Pursuit of Happyness*. He was a hardworking man, but due to circumstances found himself homeless with his two-year-old son. He could very easily have played the victim, however he made the choice not to play that card. Instead he chose to fight for his son's and his own lives, and now he is a very successful entrepreneur, investor and international inspirational speaker.

When someone says, "That person has a good attitude," the speaker means they are positive, delightful, and you want to be around them. When they pass you by, they leave a beautiful smelling perfume in their trail. On the other hand, if a person has a bad attitude, they are negative, nasty, and you just don't want to be around them. Everything is a drama or nightmare when they are around. When they pass you by, their perfume is simply and quite honestly nauseating and revolting. We all have people like that in our lives.

Where does that come from? It comes from the choices they make.

It is our responsibility to take control of our thoughts and attitude. We have the control, no one else. Next we are going to see how we can tame our thoughts to cause us to win. Win with our health, win with our relationships, win in life.

2. Your Thinking Mind and Your Thinking Heart

"If you think right, you work right."

– Dr. Amen

Why is it that some people can lose weight and keep it off, while others lose the weight and it eventually comes back? It all has to do with our thinking.

One of the contestants in *The Biggest Loser* TV show went into the competition aiming to win the whole thing. He lost 79 kg (174 lbs), but he didn't win the competition and felt like a failure. Six months later he had regained 53 kgs (116 lbs). Why? Because no one taught him how to think. Truly, if you think right, you work right.

How do we think right?

I want you to imagine a big balloon. Now imagine two big balloons. One represents your head, and the other your heart. All good so far? Next make a horizontal line across both balloons. The top part is your *conscious* (the part of you that you are aware of) and below the line is your *unconscious* (the part of you that you are not aware of – like your breathing, heart rate and temperature). The brain balloon, we will call your thinking mind. The heart balloon, we will call your thinking heart. Stay with me, we need to get the basics down before we go on with this analogy. When I was first introduced to this concept, I drew it out, and that helped me. The line that goes across the middle of your brain and heart we will call a door. And this door is always open. Whatever the top part of your brain and heart hear will also be placed in the bottom part.

So the door that connects the top to the bottom part of your brain and heart is always open, and both the brain and the heart are thinking. Now let's drop a thought like a seed into your brain and heart. All seeds (thoughts) get planted in the conscious part, and over time – since the door is always open – they take root in the subconscious part.

The soil in your brain and heart's subconscious is very obedient. Much like a farmer's field, it will grow anything you plant. If you plant a corn seed, you will get a corn plant. Equally, if you plant a seed of hemlock (which is a poison, and can kill people), then it will grow a hemlock plant. The subconscious ground cannot tell the difference between a 'good-for-you seed' like corn and a 'not-so-good-for-you seed'.

The same principle applies to our thoughts. Every thought is like a seed, and it will bear certain fruit. It can bring about a positive result or a negative result. It is your choice what you plant.

Every decision has a future attached to it. Every seed you allow to take root will bear fruit. Good seeds have good futures attached to them. Bad seeds have a bad future attached to them. We need to be very careful what we plant.

What are you planting?

Have you ever heard the saying "what you think about, comes about"? This is so true. You can always tell what people are thinking about and/or feeling because of what comes out of their mouth.

- If people choose to plant jealous seed then they talk envy.
- If people choose to plant a grateful seed then they talk joy.
- If people choose to plant the "I can do it!!!" seed then they talk about overcoming and winning.

Your chances of success are actually based on what you say to yourself. Here's a rough guide showing how what you say will affect your chances of succeeding:

- "I won't" results in 0% success
- "I can't": 10% success
- "I don't know how": 20%
- "I wish I could": 30%
- "I want to": 40%
- "I think I might": 50%
- "I might": 60%
- "I think I can": 70%
- "I can": 80%
- "I am": 90%
- "I did": 100%

The key is to plant seeds from the "I am" category, claiming who the new recreated and repositioned 'you' is – thoughts like "I am a winner", "I am diligent", "I am healthy". Do your best to reject thoughts of limitation and failure in your mind and heart, and replace them with words of victory, health, success and joy.

Making sure your mind and heart are in sync

It's important to realise that your mind and your heart are a Mastermind team. A Mastermind is a collection of harmonious co-operation of two or more, who ally themselves for the purpose of accomplishing any given task. In the business world a company like Apple has a Mastermind team to create a successful product. It is important for all members of the Mastermind team to be on the same page instead of sabotaging each other. For instance, in your head you can say "I'm going to lose weight" but your heart's thoughts are "It'll never happen". Well, guess what: the negative wins.

Another example is my 16-year-old daughter's effort to learn how to drive a manual (stick shift) car. She would tell herself she could do it, but her heart thought differently and would tell her "I can't, I'm afraid" – and she froze. After a little love and encouragement, she was able to get her mind and heart Mastermind heading in the same direction, and she passed her test and got her learner's license. Yeah!

Getting the heart and mind to move in unison toward your goal is paramount to your success in whatever you do. My recommendation is to listen to what you are thinking about, and listen to what you are saying. If they are mirroring each other, then all is good. But if they aren't, then you need to work on either your heart or your mind.

3. Forgiveness as a Cure

Imagine that someone says something insensitive to you and hurts your feelings. Or say someone promises you something, and then doesn't live up to that promise. Now, every time you see them your stomach churns, the hairs on your neck stand up, and you wish nothing but doom and gloom to happen to them.

Guess what? You have just allowed the seed of unforgiveness to take root in your subconscious soil.

What fruit is produced when we plant this seed?

- unhappiness
- anger
- victim mentality
- depression

- bitterness
- guilt
- bondage
- suppressed immune system
- frown wrinkles on our face

When we are full of unforgiveness it is as if we have drunk poison expecting it to harm the other person. We need to do ourselves a favour and save a lot of time and anger by forgiving. How do you know when you need to forgive someone more? Very easy: when you see, think, or hear that person, and you feel anger, rage or hate, then you need to keep on forgiving.

I realise that humans do some terrible things, so I am not making light of the hurts that you have suffered. I too have planted many seeds of unforgiveness. However, when I learned how unforgiveness hurts me more than it hurts the other person, I soon realised it was a losing investment.

The problem with people is that they are 'so *people*' and they don't think about what their words or actions do to us. To this day, I still have to be very aware not to allow the seed of unforgiveness to take root and grow its huge tree in my heart. The good news is that we are in control now, and we know the signs! We can pull this out by the roots – either when it's a small seedling, or when it's an enormous tree with a well entrenched root system. It's our choice.

My recommendation to you is to keep on forgiving until you don't have to forgive any more. You will know this when you see, think of or hear the person who offended you, and you feel love and peace. Yes, it may take some time, but keep at it … this too is good for your emotional health. There are people I had to forgive in my past. It's not easy sometimes, but the benefits far outweigh the nasty side effects of unforgiveness.

"Listen carefully, you need to forgive to free your own life up. When you forgive someone, you are exhibiting the most God-like character, and with it comes a peace that surpasses all understanding. Trust me, I have had to do a lot of it."
– John Maxwell, worldwide leadership authority

4. What to Say

Did you know that your life is like a blank canvas and you have the paintbrush right in your hand?

What kind of life are you painting? I hope to coach you to paint a healthy life. Painters see the picture in their minds before they actually paint it. Here is a story which demonstrates this powerful principle.

A woman who had lost 45 kg (100 lbs) was beautiful, happy and now very confident. When asked how she did it she said, "I tried diet after diet without results. The key was not to diet, but to see myself at a certain weight first." She saw herself at a particular weight in her mind's canvas, which was then painted onto her life canvas.

That brings me to my next question: What are you seeing on the inside? Are you seeing breast cancer, diabetes, even a heart attack? Are you saying "I will never get rid of this weight"? "I will always be a smoker"? You don't have to be sick! 80% of chronic disease is preventable through lifestyle changes.

You don't have to have diabetes type 2, high blood pressure, high cholesterol, cancer, and even Alzheimer's disease. Did you know that? I honestly didn't until I became a member of The Institute of Functional Medicine. It was there that I was exposed to the root cause of disease. And that's why I'm here now to bring you hope for a healthier future.

By the time I'd finished my medical training and practised medicine for 10 or so years, I just thought we gave people pills to cure them. It was a revelation when I realised that we don't have a healthcare system, we only have disease management – and I was one of those managers. I hated it. I became a doctor to help people be their best, not to manage their dis-ease.

I would like to share with you what I say to myself every day, which translates into the picture I paint for my life. The goal is to give you an idea of the sorts of statement you can make to yourself, also known as *positive affirmations*. Because what we think about, comes about:

- I am strong, toned and full of energy.
- I am getting prettier and prettier everyday (on the inside, which then radiates on the outside).
- I am safe for success.
- I am healthy.

Do you get the idea? Do you see what you can be or do you see what you can't be? You are the painter with the brush and canvas right in front of you.

Below are a few affirmations you might wish to use or add to. The purpose is to give you ideas from which you can create your own unique affirmations. That's how I did it: I built my own affirmations on the words of others.

Remember: If you can change your words, you can change your world.

Here goes:

- I am making a positive difference in people's lives.
- I am clear about my goals but I am flexible about how I achieve them.
- I believe.
- I am like a tree in the wind, I bend but I don't break.
- Success does not happen by accident.
- I am positive.
- I can do this (and I have a set of stairs going up next to the statement for a visual effect).
- Winners never quit and quitters never win.
- I am a winner.
- I become what I think about.
- My prosperity is good for all people.
- "When I have finally decided that a result is worth getting, I go ahead on it and make trial after trial until it comes." – Thomas Edison
- Whatever I passionately pursue, I will possess.
- My playing small serves no one.
- Every day and in every way I am becoming better and better.
- I don't have to believe every stupid thought that I think.
- I am an overcomer.
- Don't break…bounce.
- I love public speaking.
- I add value to people's lives.

The list can go on and on and on and…well, you know what I mean.

The bottom line, my friend, is this:

> *"Be careful how you are talking to yourself,*
> *because you are listening."*
>
> – Lisa M. Hayes

I encourage you to make a list of positive affirmations, and make them in the present tense. For instance " I am ..." or " I can ..." That way your conscious brain starts to believe what you tell it. Laminate the sayings, and put them up all over your home. You will become filled with their message. I have. Even more, you will be adding value to those who visit your home. They too will become inspired.

Like the saying goes, you can't give birth to something if you haven't conceived it. Go ahead, conceive your new repositioned life!

> *Check **www.doctoronamission.com***
> *for the upcoming date of*
> *"14-DAY WEIGHT LOSS COURSE"*
> *for your start to permanent weight loss.*

5. How to Block

In this section we will learn the technique of blocking out all thoughts that would hinder your recreated healthy self from blossoming. But before we go any further, I want to congratulate you! Yes, you. Why? Please allow me to explain.

Having a health goal should be something we all have and want to achieve. Unfortunately, we can't rely on hope or a magic pill to make us fit and healthy. We can't blame someone else for our bad health decisions, either.

We all make choices in life, and we need to take responsibility for them. You have. For that I congratulate you. Strong work.

How do we make choices?

Earlier in this book I discussed the importance of writing down your goals. Now I want to re-emphasise this, saying it in a different way, because of its importance in your success. Your success is important to me.

Here are the three steps to making a choice.

1. **Have a goal.** Having a goal makes you stronger, healthier and happier.
2. **Write your goal down.** By writing it down you are claiming that goal for yourself. The seed of that goal will germinate and take root in the sub-

conscious soil of both your mind and your heart, and produce fruit. Let me give you a recent real-life miracle illustration.

A mentor and friend of mine, Dave Bradley, author of *Build Your Team, Build Your Dream*, told me two years ago that he was in the process of writing a book. I immediately thought to myself, "I have a book inside me that I want to write!" That's what happens when you are mentored by people of integrity and vision, you begin to mirror them. There was just one problem: I didn't write down my goal to write a book. And so I really didn't mirror my mentor. It wasn't until Dave told me that his book was finished, and he sent a copy to Michael and me in New Zealand, that it hit me. I still had the goal to write a book, but I hadn't written down my goal to write a book! I woke up and wrote my goal down. Guess what? The next execution step appeared! Michael got an email from another one of our mentors, Dr. John Maxwell, author of 73 books, on … wait for it … wait for it … "A day about books and how to write a book", a webinar in June 2012. And the rest is history.

Can you see how the simple step of writing down your goal leads to the next step and then the next step and then … ? Pretty cool, isn't it!

3. **Reward yourself.** Once you have achieved your goal you need to reward yourself. You deserved it. I don't mean with food. Consider a massage, pedicure, new outfit, walking shoes, movie, etc.

If you don't reach your goal, it's ok … just reset the goal. No big deal. Progress occurs with mistakes. If you aren't failing, then you aren't moving, you are stagnant and not growing. Consider a child learning to walk. The child falls. Do you tell it to stay down? Of course not. You brush off the dirt and help it back up. Well, the same philosophy applies to you. Help yourself back up and reset the goal, my friend.

On to blocking

To become your best you need to stop listening to the wrong voices. I'm giving you permission to close the door – or, put another way, to place a block on toxic people in your life.

- Be allergic to negative people (I personally get hives when I'm around negative people).

- Be allergic to negative self talk.
- Know your enemy (which is your negative thoughts).

Remember the picture of your mind and your heart that we talked about earlier? The top part is your conscious part, the part that you are aware of. The bottom part is the subconscious part, the part that you are not aware of. Consider the bottom part, full of soil.

When a farmer plants his seeds, he prepares the ground. This is because he knows a great seed planted in soil full of weeds will not produce a great crop.

The same philosophy applies to your success. All your success begins in your mind. So let's get your soil ready for planting, shall we? Let's look at the components of your soil.

A. Faith

Faith is knowing you are created to be your best and do great things. Faith reminds us to be open to a greater power – God, higher force, The Almighty One – for the way to your goals. It is realising that it is not all up to you. All you need to be is open, teachable, and motivated to receive direction. I love the way Ralph Waldo Trine explains faith: "Faith is an invisible and invincible magnet, and attracts to it whatever it fervently desires and calmly and persistently expects."

But … you still need to put in the W O R K. Work is a good four-letter word. Which leads us to the next component of your soil.

B. Belief

Belief is the work part of faith. Belief is active, not passive. I can give you an example.

When I decided to become a doctor, I had the faith to do it. I also had to put in the work, which was me believing that I would become a doctor. You might have faith that you will lose weight and become a sexy younger you. However, as you know, that will require work. "Whoever does not doubt at all in his heart, but believes that what he says will take place, it will be done for him" Jesus says in Mark 11:23. Yes, you just "gotta believe" your goals will occur.

C. Weeds

Every farmer has to spray for weeds, knowing that a great seed planted in soil full of weeds will not produce a great crop. What kind of weeds are we talking about?

- Bitterness
- Unforgiveness
- Hatred
- Jealousy
- Greed
- Cynicism
- Doubt

Be on the alert for these weeds. They will stop you dead in your tracks and you will never reach your goal.

Ok, we have our mind and heart's soil ready with faith and belief. And we have sprayed for weeds. Now let's take a step outside our mind and heart, and see how we can protect ourselves from the outside environment.

Imagine a door. On one side of the door is you. On the other side is the world. This door can open and close. The world consists of people, and people can say positive or negative things. We can either open the door to what they say, or close the door.

I want to encourage you to open the door if it is positive, but slam it shut if it is negative. You have that power. We will call closing the door to a negative 'Blocking'. You can say it under your breath. You don't have to shout it out – people might think you're nuts.

People who love you dearly can sometimes make negative statements, and not even know it. I will use my husband Michael as an example, only to prove a point, not to pick on him. He really is my rock.

I announced to Michael that I was going to start telling a joke before I start all my public speaking engagements. I had seen other public speakers do it and found it fun. Michael's response was "Babe, you aren't good at telling jokes." Immediately in my head I said "Block". He didn't know I did it. I just did it. Now I know that Michael loves me and would do anything for me, but my point is even people who are close to you can say negative things. It is our responsibility to block those statements from access into our brain and heart.

Just shut the door. Just block it.

So access was denied, and I went on to learn how to tell a joke. Now before every speaking engagement I crack a joke, get the audience smiling, and away we go. I love it!

6. Your Mastermind Team

When you have a dream or a goal you can start small, but don't start alone. In this section I will reveal to you who is on my Mastermind team to help me succeed in reaching my dreams.

Before we start I need to prepare you.

You may think what I'm about to share with you is a little weird, but that's ok. I would prefer you to think that I'm weird rather than just a normal person. Being normal is nothing to brag about. There's nothing creative in being normal. Plus being normal is not healthy. Take a look out there in the world and see what normal is. It just isn't good.

I was reading an amazing book by Napoleon Hill called *The Laws of Success*. It took me about 16 months to complete it, because I read and applied one chapter per month. Mr. Hill helped me expand on a concept my mother taught me as a child, the concept of angels. Angels are very much a part of my invisible Mastermind team, and the Leader of my Mastermind team is God. In the Bible it says "For He shall give His angels charge over you, to keep you in all your ways. In their hands they shall bear you up, so you don't dash your foot against a stone." (Psalm 91:11–12) That's just so thoughtful of God to give us angels to help us hydroplane over the rough patches of our life so that we don't even scratch our feet.

Let me introduce you to my 11 angels, each with their own unique place on my path to success.

Patience

Patience teaches me to have composure while I wait. I am naturally a very impatient person. My husband Michael, on the other hand, is very patient. It is very helpful to see patience in action by looking at the way he handles rough spots. And it is great to have my angel Patience help me to be more like Michael.

Joy

I call my joy angel Shasta because we used to have a dog with that name. Shasta had the spirit of joy in her always, no matter what. Nothing could ever take her joy away. Shasta teaches me to enjoy this journey, not dread it.

Health

I call my health angel Doc. Doc goes to work when I go to sleep. If I am sick, or in pain before I go to bed, then I ask him to please get to work. And when I get up, I feel better and stronger and healed. Most of the time. Sometimes he has to work a double or triple shift on me.

Wisdom

Guides me to make right choices.

Financial Prosperity

Helps me do the following:
- not overspend
- set goals
- invest
- have abundant thinking

Peace of mind

Peace sings this song that you may know. I'll sing you a line … "Everything is gonna be all right, yea … cuz that's the seeds I sow … Wowowo, wowowo, wowowo wo." How was that? Peace reminds me that all I have to do is trust God and do right. Simple enough.

Hope and Faith

These two are together because you can't have one without the other. Hope tells me to never, ever, ever give up. Hope also coaches me to expect better, and better comes. Faith reminds me to worry about nothing and pray about everything.

Love and Romance

This pair cannot exist without the other. Love tells me to always believe the best and wish well for my enemies. Love also helps me develop love for *all* of humanity, because a negative attitude towards others will never bring me success. Romance adds the right mood to the whole project.

Roaming Ambassador

I call her Gwenie, another dog we used to have. But we had to put her down because she was very ill with liver cancer. Gwenie does everything else the other angels don't, like finding me a good parking spot, and letting me know about good clothing sales.

There you have my invisible Mastermind team. They are priceless and always on call for me. I am grateful for my mom and Mr. Hill for talking to me about them.

> *"Some people have a dream but no team –*
> *their dream is impossible.*
> *Some people have a dream and are building a team –*
> *their dream has potential.*
> *Some people have a dream and a great team –*
> *their dream is inevitable."*
> – Dr. John Maxwell

CHAPTER FIVE

Effective Exercise

*"It's like brushing your teeth and paying taxes…
we have to do it."* – Dr. Isabel

1. Quick Facts for Your Back Pocket

Who loves to exercise? Unfortunately it's something we have to do, just like brushing our teeth, taking a shower, and paying taxes.

Exercise can dig up some bad thoughts, like being embarrassed – maybe you were always the last one to be picked for the team – or painful memories, because of the lactic acid buildup it caused. Regardless of how we feel, we need to shake that bootie whether we're young, old, or old-young.

I like to focus on the positives. Together let's look at the benefits of effective exercise:

- Controls weight
- Promotes maximum bone density…so bones don't break as easily
- Strengthens and tones, which makes you look younger (the more muscle you have, the younger your body actually is. Yeah!)
- Enhances flexibility
- Boosts energy
- Promotes better sleep
- Improves quality of life
- Combats health conditions and diseases
- Improves mood
- Lowers blood sugar
- Lowers blood pressure

- Promotes social well-being by improving self-confidence and the ability to interact socially with peers.

It was demonstrated at the University of Colorado that modest exercise can even help prevent colds. This study found people who participated in a daily exercise programme were less likely to get sick after stressful situations. The bottom line is that we need to change our attitude about exercise. If you're still struggling with the concept of exercise, then I encourage you to change what you're saying to yourself.

Remember: if we can change our words we can change our life. Start by saying:

- I am becoming a better me.
- I feel great when I exercise.
- I can do it!
- Day by day in every way I am getting stronger and stronger.
- I may not be where I want to be, but at least I'm not where I used to be.
- I make exercise a priority.

When you reach a goal, remember to reward yourself with something nice like clothes, movie, hot bath, massage, etc.

Hope that helps.

2. Interval Training

There are three parts to effective exercise:

1. Interval training
2. Resistance training
3. Rest

Interval training is another term used to replace *cardio training*. Studies have indicated that exercise with a 'burst' component to it is more effective in helping people lose weight, especially the belly fat.

Amazingly, over-exercising can actually make us fat. When I heard this, I really felt like my brain had been scrambled. How can this occur?

Remember this diagram back in an earlier chapter:

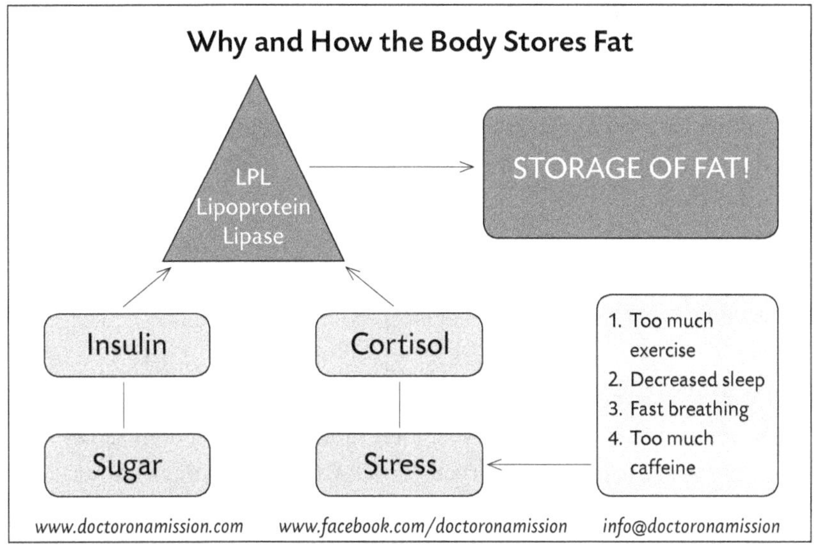

Fig 3: Why and how the body stores fat

You can see how stress raises your cortisol levels, and in the end the body stores fat. This really happened to me. Michael and I would wake up at 5am religiously and go to spin-bike class (you may know it as RPM). It is a full-on bike session for 60 minutes. The goal was to burn calories. We burned calories all right. We also gained weight, and not the good muscle kind. We were at it for one and a half years, three times a week.

Until I came across the diagram above. This made me realise that though we were burning calories and sweating up a storm, we were also stressing our bodies out. This caused cortisol to increase, resulting in storage of fat.

What did I do next? I slept in! A 5am start in the gym is just nasty. Next I started to add interval training and the weight keeps on coming off, even at my tender age of 52 years young.

The backbone of interval training is simple:

- 5–10 minutes warm up
- 5–20 minutes of a 1:2 ratio workout
- 5 minutes cool down
- 2–3 times a week

For instance: 30 seconds hard at an exercise, then recovery of 60 seconds, 6–8 repetitions. Exercise options could be biking, jogging, rowing, walking, swimming, jump rope, stairs.

Studies have found you can boost your metabolism, burn more calories all day long and lose more weight by exercising *less*. All I can say to that is a big yahoo!

You are also getting another benefit by doing interval training: because your body is not experiencing oxidative stress you won't age as quickly as you would doing other exercises that stress your body.

3. Resistance Training

Where interval training increases your metabolism to burn fat, *resistance training* has a different goal. It strengthens your muscles, which helps you burn fat all day long. This is called 'afterburn', burning fat while you are resting. It also keeps you looking and acting young.

You read right. Having more muscle makes your body younger. Conversely, having more fat is a stress on your poor body, and it ages you real fast, putting a stress load on your system *and* increasing inflammation which, as we have seen, leads to chronic disease such as hypertension, diabetes Type 2, heart disease, certain cancers and Alzheimer's disease. Having more muscle melts away the fat, and you become a lean fat-burning machine instead of a fat-storing machine.

Women do not need to do heavier weights, just the lighter weights. Rest assured, women do not bulk up because they don't have testosterone. Men, on the other hand, have testosterone and therefore bulk up with muscle. Do this 20–30 minutes per session, 2–3 times a week, and you will become 'mighty fine scenery'!

Question: How do we lose weight?

Answer: With both interval and resistance training.

Women – Just the facts

Remember: I'm just the messenger, so please don't shoot the messenger!

1. According to the *American Journal of Preventative Medicine*, a married woman who has one baby gains an average of nine kilograms (20 pounds) over ten years.

2. For every child we have, our rate of obesity increases by 7% over our lifetime. If we have three children our risk of obesity increases by 21% (Duke University Medical Center).

    Why does this happen? Pregnancy causes an increase in insulin production, which results in accumulation of fat.

3. Menopausal women have an average weight gain of five kilograms (12 pounds) within eight years after menopause. Fat burning decreases 32% due to a decrease in estrogen, according to a study in the *International Journal of Obesity*.

All the more reason for us ladies to do interval and resistance training, to stay younger and sexier.

Men – Just the facts

Same applies here … remember I'm just the messenger (big smiley face just for you)!

As you age, your testosterone levels reduce (that is the hormone that makes you all muscular and sexy). With aging there is a natural tendency for muscle to become fat. That fat likes to accumulate around the belly area, which is very dangerous. Where there is belly fat, there is an increased risk of a heart attack.

And for you, I also recommend interval and resistance training.

What about the last step, rest?

And lastly we want to rest … ahhh. Rest between workouts. You won't get results if you don't – muscles actually grow when they are resting. If you overtrain and don't rest, then your body will get tired and stressed, leading to decreased energy, increased sickness and oxidative stress. You will age faster!

EXERCISE GUIDE

1. Interval Training

- 5–10 minutes warm-up
- 1:2 ratio, for example 30 seconds hard out (puffing hard), 60 seconds slow pace (don't stop, just slow down)
- 6–8 repetitions
- Running, running up stairs, biking, jogging, walking, rowing, swimming, jumping rope.
- Approximately 20 minutes of 1:2 ratio. If you can only do 5 minutes that's fantastic. Pace yourself to get to 20 minutes. You will get there.
- 5 minutes cool down
- 2–3 times a week

2. Resistance Training

- lift some type of weight
- 20–30 minutes per day
- 2–3 times a week

3. Rest

- Alternate Interval with Resistance throughout the week, with at least one full rest day free of everything.
- Maybe on your rest day take a 45-minute walk.

CHAPTER SIX

Sugar, Obesity, and Our Future

1. My Journey with Sugar

Let's begin this chapter with a story.

A mother brought her child to see Gandhi and asked him, "Please tell my child to stop eating sugar." Gandhi said, "Bring her back in three days." Three days later the mother brings her child back to him and says: "I am confused – why did you tell me to come back in three days?" Gandhi said, "Because three days ago I was eating sugar."

I tell you this story because I know how hard it is to give up sugar. I was a sugar junkie – remember I was the doc who had a bag of candy and coffee for a strong start to my morning. Society has a sugar addiction and an overweight problem. People are bulging out of their clothes. Especially the kids.

So how did I break off my love affair with sugar? It was a decision I made when I realised that I was being tricked into eating more sugar.

I believed that in order to be healthy I needed to be on a low-fat diet. But guess what happens when you take the fat out of food? It tastes like cardboard. You also don't feel satisfied after eating. You see, eating fat is satisfying – in other words, it fills you up. So a low-fat diet replaces the satisfaction of fat with more sugar and salt.

When I learned that excess sugar gets stored as fat, the alarm bells went off. Oh it wasn't pretty in our house! I have two teenage daughters and my husband who were also addicted to sugar. The problem was they didn't realise it.

My mother has always described me as a pioneer and courageous. I went through our cupboards and refrigerator and began reading labels. The more I read, the madder I got, and the fuller the trash bin grew.

I have a saying: "Waking up is very painful." It's painful to face reality because we get comfortable in our routines – like the routine of going to do groceries, and buying the same cereal week after week after week. Until one day you wake up, begin reading the label, and find some form of sugar within the first five ingredients. I just got mad when I realised I was poisoning my family and affecting their health. But before I was able to talk the talk, I had to walk the talk. So I went on a sugar fast. It was ugly!

For one whole month I didn't allow one drop of any type of sugar past my lips. The only sweet things that made it into my mouth were 1–2 low-GI pieces of fruit per day, such as:

- grapefruit
- kiwi
- coconut
- strawberries
- apple
- avocado
- any berry
- plum
- green grapes
- cherries

It's mindblowing to taste the natural sweetness in fruit!

The withdrawal symptoms I went through as I went cold turkey on sugar were those experienced by any addict coming off their drug of choice. Headaches, sugar and carb craving, joint pain, fatigue, loss of clarity of thinking, and low moods. The only withdrawal I was spared was the sweating. But the good news is, the symptoms go away, and so does some weight!

I bet you're wondering if I ever eat sugar. That's like asking me if the pope is Catholic. There are times when I just go for it and have sugar. I'm a human being! But the difference now is that it doesn't go on day after day, year after year.

Back to my family. After my own month of withdrawal, I had the right heart attitude to deal with my family's sugar withdrawal. So I put them on a sugar detox. How? I just stopped bringing sugared foods into the home. No more ice cream, cereal, tomato sauce, cookies, cakes, jams, lunchbox snacks, chips, sauces, on and on and on. I'm glad to say we are still all alive and living under the same roof. My family really loved the weight loss side effect too. Yes, we do have treats, but now they're very limited. After all, I want to stay alive.

If you're the person who brings the food into the home, I encourage you to do as Gandhi did and stop eating sugar. Then you will better understand and guide your family through the tough times of removing sugar (well, at least 80% of it) from their lives,.

Below is a list of places sugar hides. I know I showed this in a previous chapter, but it's worth repeating – I really believe having this information will add value to your life and those you come in contact with.

Places where sugar hides

- Agave syrup or agave sugar. Yes, agave has a low-GI profile, but what it does is actually far worse than raising insulin levels: it raises your triglyceride levels, triggers inflammation and damages your liver.
- Barley malt
- Beet sugar
- Brown sugar
- Buttered syrup
- Cane juice crystals
- Cane sugar
- Caramel
- Corn syrup
- Corn syrup solids
- Confectioner's sugar
- Carob syrup
- Castor sugar
- Date sugar
- Demerara sugar
- Dextran
- Dextrose
- Diastatic malt
- Diatese
- Dried fruit (high-GI, and all just concentrated sugar)
- Ethyl Maltol
- Fructose

- Fruit juice
- Fruit juice concentrate
- Galactose
- Glucose
- Glucose solids
- Golden sugar
- Golden syrup
- Grape sugar
- High-Fructose Corn Syrup (HFCS)
- Sugar of maize
- Honey
- Icing sugar
- Invert sugar
- Lactose
- Maltodextrin
- Maltose
- Malt syrup
- Maple syrup
- Molasses
- Muscovado sugar
- Panocha
- Raw sugar
- Refiner's sugar
- Rice syrup
- Sorbitol
- Sorghum syrup
- Sucrose
- Sugar
- Treacle
- Turbinado sugar
- Yellow sugar
- and finally, anything ending in '-ose' is sugar.

You now have your PhD in 'sugar disguises'. Now the question arises, "What can I use as a sweetener?" I always recommend stevia. Stevia is a plant from the sunflower family and is 300 times sweeter than sugar. Stevia is a low-GI food and if you need something as a sweetener then stevia is your best option. This is what we use in our family. I personally prefer the stevia drops as opposed to the powder, as I can control the sweetness more readily.

I promise you that once you remove all of the above from your life, the foods that you do eat will taste sweet. You can do this. Plus, as a bonus, you will instantly lose some weight.

2. The Bitter Truth

Dr. Lustig, a paediatrician at The University of San Francisco, USA, has put together a lecture called *The Bitter Truth* which I encourage you to view on YouTube. He is on a mission to end obesity and diabetes in our youth. I am in complete agreement with this.

The old thinking was that patients go to their doctor to lose weight. The doctor supplies the following equation:

Eat less + Eat a low-fat diet + Exercise more = Weight loss

When the patients come back without losing weight, the doctor thinks they are lazy gluttons with no willpower. The poor patient gets the same prescription again, but this time with a diet pill:

Diet pill + Eat less + Eat a low-fat diet + Exercise more

Perhaps they lose a bit of weight when the diet pill is added, but over time the weight comes back – with a few more kilos on top! The argument that children are lazy gluttons just doesn't stand either. No child chooses to be obese. They just eat what they are given. Indeed, no one chooses to be obese!

I have been a doctor for 22 years, and all I can say is *"This doesn't work!"*

Yes, we are eating more, but that is not the reason why ⅔ of America, UK, Australia and NZ is overweight – *and* ⅓ of those are obese. Mark Twain said so eloquently, "Education consists mainly of what we have unlearned." We need to rethink the equation and unlearn what we have learned.

In the past we have focused on BMI (Body Mass Index) as an indicator of weight, where:

- less than 19 BMI = underweight
- 20–25 BMI = healthy

- 26–29 BMI = overweight
- greater than 30 = obese

We need to unlearn this and relearn the new. The new measurement is our waist size. New research indicates that the goal is to have your waist size less than half of your height.

For instance, if you are 170 cm, then ideally your waist should be less than 85 cm. Alternatively, if you are 72 inches (6 ft), then your waist circumference should be 36 inches or less.

A new study by Dr. Amen of the Amen Clinics in USA concludes: "An increase in the size of your waist leads to a decrease in the size of your brain." So the bigger your waist, the smaller your brain. Now that should scare everyone into losing those unhealthy love handles!

Does diet and exercise work? No. Exercising past a certain point stresses the body, causing it to store fat for future energy needs. Exercise is not the answer.

Looking at behaviour

What makes us obese?

There are many reasons why there is so much obesity all around us in the western world. What surrounds us has the most impact.

- Food is available to us 24 hours per day, seven days a week.
- Food tastes really good. Food companies put in food enhancers to make food smell and taste good. I had a patient go into Burger King for a meal. He said it "tasted good while ,I was eating it, but boy it's painful when it lands!" The reason he was in to see me was because he had diarrhoea the next day and needed an off-work certificate.
- There are more TV food commercials. Count the number of food commercials you see next time you are watching TV. The average child sees 10,000 ads for junk food on TV in one year. American Idol has judges with Coke cups in front of them.
- Grocery stores have all the sugar products on the lower shelves. This is purposely done so our children can see them.
- There is something in our diet called High-Fructose Corn Syrup (HFCS), which we will address shortly.

- In 1980 we were advised to decrease fat and increase our sugar consumption by eating more carbs. We now know this didn't work. As I have mentioned before, when you take the fat out of food you need to make it taste better, and that was accomplished by adding HFCS.

Bottom line? We're influenced by what we see and smell.

3. High-Fructose Corn Syrup

In the past 30 years, our percentage of sugar calories from High-Fructose Corn Syrup (HFCS) has increased from 0% to 66%. This, sadly, is due to our consumption of soft drinks and other sweetened beverages. We also know that liquid calories in the form of sugar pack on the weight.

What is HFCS?

HFCS is an industrial food product – not a natural food, nor a whole food. Extracted from corn stalks by a chemical process, it is sweeter than sugar. It is also cheaper, and so is used more readily.

What does it do to your body?

This compound is rapidly absorbed into your bloodstream and sent to your liver. Once in the liver, a reaction called lipogenesis (the production of fats like triglycerides and cholesterol) occurs. Your liver gets taxed from overwork, and this is the major cause of liver damage, also known as fatty liver. In addition, because it is so rapidly absorbed, there is a spike in your insulin. What we know of to date is that these two features of HFCS increase appetite, weight gain, diabetes, heart disease and dementia.

HFCS also affects your gut. Connections in your intestine between the intestinal cells are called 'tight junctions'. They have one main dual purpose: to allow nutrients in, and prevent bacteria and other not-so-healthy food compounds from getting through. If the bacteria make it through these 'tight junctions', this triggers an immune response of body-wide inflammation.

HFCS creates exactly this situation by punching holes in the intestinal lining of the gut. This allows the enemy in, and fullscale war breaks out in your gut. You may have heard of this referred to as 'Leaky Gut Syndrome'; HFCS is one cause.

What does HFCS contain?

An American FDA researcher asked corn producers to ship a barrel of high-fructose corn syrup to her so that she could test for contaminants. Her repeated requests were denied until she claimed she represented a newly created soft drink company. She was then promptly shipped a big vat of HFCS, which was used in a study showing that HFCS often contains toxic levels of mercury, due to the chlor-alkali products used in its manufacture.

The companies that produce HFCS often say in TV ads that HFCS is exactly like sugar. I want you to realise one thing: poisoned sugar, like that created in the production of HFCS, is certainly not natural.

Real sugar consists of glucose and fructose. When HFCS is placed through a chemical analyser, strange peaks show up that do not coincide with the normal glucose and fructose peaks. We don't really know what it is, and the producers of HFCS don't really want to share their recipe. To think that 20% of the western world is consuming this poison is not only disturbing, but frightening.

Do we need HFCS in our diets?

If you go to the friendly, happy looking websites of the corn industry (www.cornsugar.com and www.sweetsurprise.com), they say they take the same view as nutritional experts. But they misquote those nutritional experts.

Barry M. Popkins PhD, Professor, Department of Nutrition, University of North Carolina at Chapel Hill, has published widely on the dangers of sugar-sweetened drinks and their contribution to the international obesity epidemic. In a review of HFCS in the *American Journal of Clinical Nutrition*, he explains the mechanism by which free fructose may contribute to obesity. He states that:

"The digestion, absorption, and metabolism of fructose differ from those of glucose. Hepatic metabolism of fructose favors de novo lipogenesis. In addition, unlike glucose, fructose does not stimulate insulin secretion or enhance leptin production. Because insulin and leptin act as key afferent signals in the regulation of food intake and body weight (to control appetite), this suggests that dietary fructose may contribute to increased energy intake and weight gain. Furthermore, calorically sweetened beverages may enhance caloric overconsumption."

Dr. Popkin concludes by saying that "the increase in consumption of HFCS has a temporal relation to the epidemic of obesity, and the overconsumption of HFCS in calorically sweetened beverages may play a role in the epidemic of obesity."

However the corn industry has taken his comments out of context to support their position that "all sugar is the same".

Here is a short biochemistry lesson about cane sugar and HFCS.

- Cane sugar is sucrose, comprising 50% fructose and 50% glucose.

  Sucrose (cane sugar) = 50% fructose + 50% glucose

- HFCS is different: it comprises 45% fructose and 55% glucose

  HFCS = 45% fructose + 55% glucose

Because glucose is sweeter than fructose, HFCS is sweeter than naturally occurring cane sugar. So the corn industry's claim that "all sugar is the same" is false.

HFCS is not a naturally occurring substance. HFCS is extracted from corn stalks and mysteriously processed as discussed in Michael Pollan's book *The Omnivore's Dilemma.*

True, large doses of any sugar are harmful, and in the end it might be the pharmacologic doses of any type of sugar that kill you. But the biochemistry of cane sugar and HFCS and how it affects our absorption, our appetite, and our metabolism are different. And Dr. Popkin knows that.

Does the presence of HFCS in food indicate an inferior quality, nutrient-poor, disease-creating food product?

Yes. If you find "High-fructose corn syrup", or the terms "corn sugar" or "sugar of maize" on the label, you can be sure it is not a whole, real, fresh food, full of fibre, vitamins and minerals.

In summary, I highly recommend that you reduce your overall consumption of sugar. However, cutting out HFCS alone will radically reduce your health risks and improve your overall health.

"To be forewarned is to be forearmed."

4. Is Diet Food Making You Fat?

Along with the beginning of the low-fat revolution came the use of artificial sweeteners. Everyone was told to eat low-fat foods and drink diet drinks. That's what I was taught in medical school. That was all the information I had to offer my patients. I have learned differently, and I want to share with you some very interesting information regarding artificial sweeteners.

To start with, we need to understand why we eat.

What drives the desire to eat?

Eating food gives us satisfaction, and shares the same brain circuitry with other pleasurable activities such as sex and drug administration. We call this food reward.

Food reward has two roads: one to the brain, and the other away from the brain.

The road to the brain is called the sensory road. When we eat there are signals that go to our brain to tell us we just ate something. Another road leaves the brain to tell our gut that we have received enough food and we are full. This is called the postingestive road.

When rats are deprived of food, then given a choice between glucose (which has 15 calories per teaspoon in it) and saccharin (which has no calories), they prefer the glucose. It appears that the artificial sweetener does not send a message along the postingestive pathway to the gut telling it "You are full".

Another study at Purdue University's Ingestive Behavior Research Center reported that relative to rats that ate yoghurt sweetened with glucose (which has calories), rats given yoghurt sweetened with 0-calorie saccharin later:

- consumed more calories
- gained more weight
- put on more body fat
- and didn't make up for it by cutting back on consumption.

Put more succinctly in the Yale Journal of Biology and Medicine, "lack of completed satisfaction, likely because of the failure to activate the postingestive component, further fuels the food seeking." So those who use artificial sweeteners are never full and keep eating.

I realise that this is all done on rats and not on humans, but the findings match emerging evidence that people who drink more diet drinks are at higher risk of obesity. They are also at risk of developing metabolic syndrome, a collection of medical problems such as abdominal fat, high blood pressure and insulin resistance that puts people at risk of heart disease and diabetes.

So if you think that diet soft drinks are the answer to weight loss, I strongly encourage you to think again. Evidence is mounting that they lead to weight gain rather then weight loss. Those who consume diet drinks regularly have a 200 percent increased risk of weight gain and a 67 percent increased risk of diabetes. One study of over 400 people found that those who drank two diet sodas per day experienced five times the increase in waist circumference of those who did not drink soda.

What are the names of artificial sweeteners?

- Nutrasweet
- Splenda
- Acesulfame potassium Ace K
- Aspartame
- Cyclamate
- Isomalt
- Saccharin
- Sucralose
- Alitame
- Neohesperidine dihydrochalcone
- Aspartame-acesulfame salt
- Sorbitol
- Maltitol

If you need something sweet, then as I have said earlier, I recommend stevia, which comes from the sunflower family, is low-GI and is 300 times sweeter than sugar. I personally don't like the aftertaste, but it's the safest natural sweetener out there.

5. What is Diabesity?

When you go to the doctor to have your blood checked, they normally do a screening test to check for Type 2 diabetes. This test, currently, is called a HgA1c (haemoglobin A1c). If your test result is under a certain number, then you are told that you don't have Type 2 diabetes. But if it's over a certain number, you *are* considered to have Type 2 diabetes.

The problem with this approach is that Type 2 diabetes doesn't happen over a month or a year. It actually starts much earlier – years, even decades earlier. You've already travelled a long journey before you ever get the dreaded diagnosis of Type 2 diabetes.

The various markers before a diabetes diagnosis is confirmed come with different names such as:

- Insulin Resistance
- Metabolic Syndrome
- Syndrome X
- Obesity
- Pre-diabetes
- Adult-onset diabetes
- Type 2 diabetes

All of these are essentially one problem. Mark Hyman MD, author of *The Blood Sugar Solution*, coins a more comprehensive term to describe the continuum from optimal blood sugar to insulin resistance to full-blown diabetes: *diabesity*. In short, diabesity is the road one is on whose final destination is Type 2 diabetes.

Diabesity (mild insulin resistance > obesity > Type 2 diabetes) is the single biggest global health epidemic of our time. It is the leading cause of chronic disease such as heart disease, stroke, dementia, and cancer. But these are all preventable diseases. You don't have to have them!

We know what the root of the problem is. "As physicians, we are trained to offer medication or surgery to solve diabetes (and disease in general), when the real causes include poor-quality diet, nutritional deficiencies, hormonal imbalances, allergens, microbes, digestive imbalances, toxins, cellular energy problems, and stress. We think that treating the risk factors, such as high blood pressure, high blood sugar, cholesterol, with medications will help. But we don't learn how to identify and treat the *real* causes of disease," says Dr. Hyman.

We need to ask the most important questions:

- Why is your blood sugar high?
- Why is your blood pressure high?
- Why is your cholesterol high?

The bottom line is, Type 2 diabetes and elevated blood sugar, blood pressure and cholesterol are symptoms resulting from problems with diet, lifestyle, and environmental toxins. By 2020 one of every two people will have diabesity, and 90% will not know it, because it is not being taught about in medical schools. Doctors don't even know how to test for it.

This is not just an adult problem, it is a childhood tragedy. We are now seeing eight year old children with Type 2 diabetes (which in the past was called 'adult onset diabetes'). Fifteen year olds with Type 2 diabetes are having strokes, and twenty-five year olds are requiring cardiac bypass. This is shocking. This is the first generation of children in history that will live sicker and die younger than their parents.

"From 1983 to 2008, the number of people in the world with diabetes increased sevenfold, from 35 to 240 million. In just three years, from 2008 to 2011, we added another 110 million diabetics to our global population," states Dr. Hyman. He adds (and I agree), "Shouldn't the main question we ask be, Why is this happening, instead of what new drug can we find to treat it? Our approach must be novel, innovative, and widely applicable at low cost across all borders." Too many billions of dollars have been spent trying to find the right drug cure.

What I hope I have done is show you that the solution is right under our nose – our mouth, and what we put into it. This is a lifestyle and environmental disease and will not be cured by medication.

Let's wake up, rise up and take back our health – for our sake and (more importantly) for our children's lives.

6. What Can We Do?

One of the most important take-home messages for you today is to know that you are in control, if you choose to be in control. If you do, then you can experience what it is like to feel clean, full of energy and have that glow that healthy people exude. If you choose not to take control of your health because it's too hard, then I recommend you go to the hospital and volunteer and care for those who chose likewise. I pray that someday you wake up.

The most challenging step for the majority of us is giving up sugar. The reason you need to give up all types of sugar is because it spikes your insulin. Type 2 diabetes develops in the presence of too much insulin. The question we want to ask is: Why is there so much insulin around? The answer is: Because there is so much sugar around.

So let's get rid of the root of the problem seen in Type 2 diabetes – sugar. Remember, when there is too much insulin around, then insulin will store sugar away as fat … especially belly fat. You want to avoid that.

Give yourself about a month to detox from sugar and you will see your waist circumference decrease, your weight come off, and your energy levels increase. Promise.

SIX SIMPLE STEPS FOR KICKING SUGAR CRAVINGS

1. Avoid sugar foods

Sugar and processed foods can be as addictive as heroin. Eating sugar artificially stimulates a region in your brain called the 'nucleus accumbens' which produces *dopamine*, the pleasure hormone. Soon dopamine levels drop and we start to feel 'flat' or a bit down. So we grab for more sugar, and round and round and up and down we go. We crave this pleasant, feel-good emotion again … so *sugar leads to addiction*.

2. Boost your serotonin

Serotonin is known as your "happy hormone", and it can be increased by:

- eating a low-GI diet as explained in Chapter 1 "What do I eat, Doc?"
- 8–9 hours of good sleep
- regular exercise

When you have sufficient serotonin, you are less likely to crave sweets.

3. Use stevia to satisfy your sweet tooth

Stevia is a natural sweetener, has no calories, won't spike your blood sugar levels, and is 300 times sweeter than sugar. It does have an aftertaste though. Stevia comes in powder and liquid form and can be purchased at a health food store.

4. Drink plenty of water

Sometimes when you think you're hungry, you're actually thirsty. Try water with five drops of stevia and a squeeze of lemon, lime or orange.

5. Keep your blood sugars stable

To avoid dips in your blood sugar eat a combination of a carbohydrate, fat and protein every four hours at each sitting. Try a celery stick or wholemeal cracker with organic almond butter or organic peanut butter for a snack.

6. Have plenty of vegetables ready

Green veggies help boost your energy and reduce cravings for sugar and processed foods. Have some always chopped up and ready to eat in the refrigerator. Try juicing your veggies for a super-charged nutrient boost. Juicing gives you a super fantastic way to add lifegiving nutrients and detoxifying plant chlorophyll to your blood stream.

WHAT DOESN'T WORK

We also need to look at what just doesn't work. In the past, public campaigns and government guidelines have been tried – for instance, warnings on cigarette product labels, or school-based education programmes tackling alcohol abuse. Yet people still continue to smoke, and we still have an incredible amount of binge drinking amongst our teenagers.

These approaches don't work because our brains have been hijacked by advertising. For every logical advertisement about the dangers of cigarettes and alcohol, there are two to three times more showing how sexy and cool it is to drink and smoke. Young people want to be accepted. Guess which ads win?

What I do know is this: Sugar is addictive like nicotine, alcohol, cannabis, morphine, amphetamine, cocaine and heroin. And we have a food war upon us. What is good for the food companies (producing cheap non-food that makes a good profit) is bad for us. I don't recommend this, but the message is clear…if you want to make money, then invest in fast food.

Addiction is not only a personal responsibility, but also a social and governmental one. Just saying "No" is not the answer. It's bigger than this. It would be fantastic if we could make a drug to stop sugar addiction, but there's no possible way from a chemical point of view.

Are you familiar with Pottenger's experiment with cats? This is an old experiment that has been repeated multiple times. Pottenger fed different groups of cats raw food and dead food. After eating dead food the cats were extinct in four generations – but the raw food cats were thriving, with healthy fur and skin.

What do people eat today? They are eating dead food.

People don't want to be obese. Children don't want to be obese. It happens because their bodies are starved of real, whole, nutrient-dense food, so they continue to eat hoping to feed their hungry bodies. Sadly, they just keep getting dead, nutrient-deficient food.

WHAT NEEDS TO WORK

Since we are influenced by what we see and hear, we need controls on advertising. Advertising the toys at McDonalds is one of the indirect ways kids are induced to eat more fast food. We need to be more like Norway, Sweden, UK and 46 other countries around the world which ban advertising to children.

A tax such as a Soda Tax would also help to decrease consumption. As with cigarette taxes in many parts of the world, we know that increasing the cost of a product decreases its use.

We should also compel fast food chains to pay a certain amount yearly to a country's medical costs. Since they are contributing to the tsunami of obesity and diabetes, they should help pay for its effects. If the food chain has a product that diminishes health then it needs to be held accountable. This will help pay for the enormous costs of obesity and the chronic diseases associated with it.

On the other hand, if a food chain adds value to a country, then the opposite should occur, and they could be given a tax break. This approach would encourage other entrepreneurs to create food companies that help heal the world. They would be adding to the solution, not the problem.

There should be restrictions on consumption. For instance, why are corner stores a few meters from schools? Maybe there should be a restriction on sales of sugar products from 3–6pm.

At doctoronamission.com, we are in the process of forming health teams to teach and guide schools and corporations about nutrition. I have found that everyone needs help understanding the rules of the body and its needs. When we can affect one person, one school, one corporation, then they will affect their world. Like the biblical saying goes: "One can put a thousand to flight, two can put ten thousand to flight." (Deuteronomy 32:30)

Can you envision what 200 can do? If our teams can work with the CEO of a home, which is usually the one who buys the food, then they will change the world of their home for this generation and generations to come. It all starts with one. Just look at what Mother Teresa and Gandhi have done.

I'm looking to join forces with big thinkers. If you have any new ideas, please contact me at: *info@doctoronamission.com*

> *Check **www.doctoronamission.com***
> *for the upcoming date of*
> ***"YOUR 14-DAY WEIGHT LOSS COURSE"***
> *for your start to permanent weight loss.*

CHAPTER SEVEN

Putting It All Together
Living a Super-Fantastic Life without Disease

1. Eating Your Medicine

We have been led to believe that if we eat whatever we want, we can counteract that with exercising. There is nothing further from the truth. There are 32-year-olds who did just that, and are having heart attacks.

Take Home Life Lesson: You can't out-train a bad diet ...

You have come this far and you are now well equipped to walk your journey back to health. There are just a few basics you need to keep in mind.

First, your medicine is at the end of your fork

You truly are what you eat. If you eat dead food, you will feel dead. If you eat live food, you will feel alive. It is as simple as that.

If you can buy organic food, go for it. If you can't, then your next best alternative is to make sure you wash your fruits and vegetables in one part white vinegar to ten parts water. Swish them around and rinse them with water. This will help remove the pesticides that reside underneath the skin.

Second, drink your water

Your body is 75% water. So many times my patients have come in saying "I feel so tired." When I ask how much water they drink, they will tell me one to two bottles. That's about 500–750 ml of water, and it's not enough. The goal is to drink at least 30 ml of water for every kg of your weight. Or if you are working in pounds, one ounce of water for every pound of weight.

70 kg person x 30 ml/kg = 2.1 litres of water per day

154 lb person x 1 ounce/lb = 154 ounces (or 1 gallon) of water per day

Make sure you don't drink your daily quota all in one sitting, as that is dangerous. Divide your daily ration into thirds and consume throughout the day.

Third, follow the food pyramid chart in Chapter 1 Section 2

This will become second nature to you after a while. You also have a list of low-to-high-GI foods in Chapter 1 Section 4: "What do I eat, Doc?"

"The best way to break a bad habit
is to replace it with a good one."

You can do it. I know you can.

2. Maximizing Your Health with Supplementation

Several of my patients ask me why they need vitamins and supplementation if they are already eating real, whole foods. Great question.

Supplements help fill in any gaps in your daily eating, when you are unable to get your requirements of micronutrients. Additionally, if we:

- lived in a world that was free of toxins
- ate only 100% real food
- were stress free
- exercised regularly
- relaxed when we needed to relax
- slept 8–9 hours every night
- drank our required amount of water, and
- had good strong healthy relationships

then I could responsibly say to you that you don't need vitamins and supplements. However, that is not the world we live in.

Here is a basic plan of what my family and I take. I personally have a few more on top of this for my specific needs.

Multivitamin/Multimineral

Many multivitamins/multiminerals offer a broad spectrum formula, ideal for everyday use to support a balanced diet. However, not all contain the following, so make sure you are getting these:

- *Zinc* and *selenium* help to support a healthy immune system
- *Vitamin B* assists with healthy brain function and energy production
- *Folic acid* assists in the maintenance of a healthy cardiovascular system and maintains normal homocysteine levels. Homocysteine is a marker of cardiovascular health.

Omega-3 Fatty Acid

I can't say enough about the importance of eating good fats, and Omega-3 is king among healthy fats.

Your body needs the right type of fats – without them it just breaks down. Every single cell in your body is made up of essential fats – yes, fats make up the wall of every single cell in your precious glorious body. (See Chapter 1 Section 4: "What do I eat, Doc?")

Omega-3s help maintain healthy insulin levels, help you avoid excessive inflammation, and help maintain healthy cholesterol levels. I encourage you to purchase good clean Omega-3s free of contaminants such as mercury. Remember, you get what you pay for, so cheap is not always good.

You need to take 1,000–2,000 mg of Omega-3 fats per day (containing a ratio of approximately 300 mg of EPA and 200 mg of DHA), once with breakfast and once with dinner.

For those on a blood thinner such as coumadin or warfarin, there is an interaction between the two which will increase your INR. Please make sure to let your doctor know whenever you are taking any supplement.

Vitamin D3

Vitamin D3 has recently been found to be lacking in a majority of people, and that lack is at the root of several diseases. In the next section you will read about Vitamin D3.

Magnesium

Diets low in magnesium are associated with increased levels of insulin and we often see magnesium deficiency in diabetics. Magnesium helps glucose enter the cells and turn those calories into energy for the body.

Magnesium is also used for the relief of muscular cramps, spasms and migraines. So I recommend this over nonsteroidal anti-inflammatories (NSAID) like:

- aspirin
- celecoxib (Celebrex)
- diclofenac (Voltaren)
- diflunisal (Dolobid)
- etodolac (Londine)
- ibuprofen (Motrin)
- indomethacin (Indocin)
- ketoprofen (Orudis)
- ketorolac (Toradol)
- nabumetone (Relafen)
- naproxen (Aleve, Naprosyn)
- oxaprozin (Daypro)
- proxicam (Feldene)
- salsalate (Amigesic)
- sulindac (Clinoril)
- tolmetin (Tolectin)

as it is easier on the gut and safer.

Diarrhoea is often a sign that you are getting too much magnesium. If this occurs just decrease the dose or switch to magnesium glycinate. You want to avoid magnesium carbonate, sulfate, gluconate, or oxide. These are the cheapest and most common forms of magnesium found in supplements, and are poorly absorbed.

If you tend to be constipated, then I recommend magnesium citrate.

N.B. People with kidney disease or severe heart disease should take magnesium only under a doctor's supervision.

3. Vitamin D3

How is Vitamin D3 produced?

Your skin makes Vitamin D3 when exposed to a 'pinking dose' of sunlight. How much vitamin D3 you will make depends on your age, how much skin is uncovered and your skin tone. The darker your skin is, the more sun you need to make enough Vitamin D3.

Sunlight exposure is the main source of Vitamin D3 for most people. However, there is no scientifically validated safe level of sun exposure. This makes recommendations regarding sun exposure difficult – one needs to weigh the risk of skin damage and skin cancer against the risk of Vitamin D3 deficiency.

Children and Vitamin D3

Dr. Cameron Grant, a New Zealand-born paediatrician, has investigated the health of children in New Zealand and discovered the sad truth about their nutritional status. Approximately 14% of New Zealand infants aged 6–23 months are iron deficient: double the rate in Australia, the US and Europe. And 10% of New Zealand children aged under two have a Vitamin D3 deficiency. A quarter of Pacifica children are Vitamin D3 deficient. (Remember: the darker your skin is, the more sun you need to make enough Vitamin D3.)

What are the results of Vitamin D3 deficiency? We are seeing children suffering from rickets, which can cause bowed legs and knocked knees. Some children are also presenting with muscle spasms and convulsions because their calcium levels are so low. This occurs because they don't have enough Vitamin D3 to help absorb the calcium.

Vitamin D3 also maintains a healthy immune function. A *vitamin deficiency* leads to more pneumonia (which is an infection in the lungs).

Adults and Vitamin D3

Vitamin D3 is essential for absorbing calcium in the gut, and so helps reduce the risk of fractures in the elderly.

Below is a list of conditions associated with certain Vitamin D3 levels. I show you this because it is important for you to see what can happen to your health if your Vitamin D3 levels are not in the optimal range.

Levels of Vitamin D3 conditions
- < 10 ng/ml: Severely deficient
- < 15 ng/ml: Risk of rickets
- < 20 ng/ml: 75% greater risk of colon cancer
- < 30 ng/ml: Deficient –
  · Increased calcium loss from bones, osteoporosis
  · Poor wound healing
  · Increased muscle pain
  · Increased joint and back pain
  · Greater risk of depression
  · Increased diabetes
  · Increased schizophrenia
  · Increased migraines
  · Increased autoimmune disease (lupus, scleroderma)
  · Increased allergies
  · Increased preeclampsia during pregnancy
  · Increased inflammation
- < 34 ng/ml: Twice the risk of heart attacks
- < 36 ng/ml: Increased incidence of high blood pressure
- <100 ng/ml: Increased risk of toxic symptoms (hypercalcemia)

Positives of Higher Levels of Vitamin D3
- 50 ng/ml: 50% reduction in breast cancer, decreased risk of all solid cancers
- 80–100ng/ml: Slowing of cancer growth in patients with cancer

The Human Warranty

"We are born with a 70 year warranty, however we never bother to read the instructions. People break down because of owner abuse and neglect, which the usual warranty doesn't cover. Upkeep is the owner's responsibility. That involves a minimum amount of regular use and the right kind of fuel."

– Dr. George Sheehan, cardiologist, runner and writer

A Quiz

Below is a little quiz you can take to get an overall idea of your Vitamin D3 levels without having to have your blood tested. If you answer yes to any of the questions, give yourself 1 point.

- Do you work indoors?
- Do you hardly ever go outside?
- Do you wear sunblock most of the time?
- Do you have the winter blues, also known as *Seasonal Affective Disorder* (SAD)?
- Do you suffer from depression?
- Do you have dark skin (any race other than Caucasian)?
- Do you rarely (or never) eat small fatty fish such as mackerel, herring or sardines (the main sources of dietary Vitamin D3)?
- Do your muscles feel sore and weak?
- Do your bones feel tender (press on your shin bone – if it hurts, you are low in Vitamin D3)?
- Do you have osteoarthritis (osteoarthritis is a result of low Vitamin D3 levels, resulting in weakened bones and thinning of bone structure)?
- Do you have osteoporosis?
- Have you broken more than two bones or fractured your hip?
- Do you suffer from mental fogginess or memory loss?
- Do you have autoimmune disease (for example lupus, multiple sclerosis, scleroderma)?
- Do you have frequent infections (colds, skin, or chest infections)?

If you scored less than 3, you are in the adequate Vitamin D3 range.

If you scored 4 or greater, then see below for sources of Vitamin D3 . I also recommend you see your physician to have your Vitamin D3 levels checked.

Points about sunblock and vitamin D3:

- We know that Vitamin D3 comes from sunlight, however so does skin cancer.
- Without sunblock and with arms and legs exposed, your skin will make 10,000 to 15,000 units of Vitamin D3 on average in one sun exposure. Most people require an additional 2,000 to 5,000 units of Vitamin D3 a day.

- Sunblock with an SPF of more than 15 blocks 100% of Vitamin D3 production in the skin.

My recommendation, supported by Dr. Mark Hyman, author of *The Blood Sugar Solution,* is the following: as well as taking a supplement of Vitamin D3, the best way to ensure adequate blood levels is to get 15 minutes of full-body sun exposure without sunscreen (although I recommend sunscreen on your face) between 10am and 2pm. This works only in the summer, which is why I recommend you take additional Vitamin D3 to optimise your level.

Other food sources of Vitamin D3 can be found in:

- Mackerel, herring, sardines
- Porcini or shiitake mushrooms
- Cod liver oil.

How to check your official levels of Vitamin D3

After reviewing the literature, you need to get your Vitamin D3 levels checked with the correct test. Ask to have your 25-OH Vitamin D levels checked. The goal is to get your blood levels up to 45–60 ng/ml. I recommend you have your Vitamin D3 levels rechecked within two weeks to two months after starting supplementation, and then yearly.

Here are the Vitamin D3 Supplementation Doses

Normal dosing of Vitamin D3 depends on your blood levels. Treatment doses (as recommended by The Institute of Functional Medicine) for blood level ranges are:

- <20 ng/ml: take 10,000 units per day
- 20–30 ng/ml: take 8,000 units per day
- 30–40 ng/ml: take 5,000 units per day
- 40–50 ng/dl: take 2,000 units per day

If you are taking a Vitamin D3 supplement, adequate calcium and magnesium intake are also required. It is very difficult to get too much Vitamin D3. People can take up to 10,000 units per day for six months and not have any adverse effects. However, people with sarcoidosis, tuberculosis, Lyme disease, lymphoma or kidney disease have to be supplemented carefully because of increased risk of their blood calcium level becoming too high.

> *If you are interested in further information regarding Vitamin D3, then I warmly invite you to come join us at www.doctoronamission.com or www.facebook.com/purelifestyle1.*

4. 12 Steps to Health and Permanent Weight Loss

We have come to the final section. To finish off, I always like to have simple guidelines to follow after I have read a book. Below are twelve steps to guide you on the road to your best health, and your permanent weight loss.

Remember, the best way to break a bad habit is to replace it with a good one. Be gentle with yourself, and know that failing is all part of the journey. When you do fall, stumble, or just crash and burn…I want you to first forgive yourself, and second dust yourself off, and get back on your road to better health.

— 12 STEPS —

1. Eat a **carbohydrate + protein + fat** every 3–4 hours. This helps keep your blood sugar stable.

2. Eat **30 to 60 minutes** after getting up. This gets your metabolism working right away.

3. Eat **low- to medium-GI foods.** This will keep your insulin from spiking, so you won't store belly fat.

4. **Avoid all processed foods.** Eat only foods your great great grandmother would recognise.

5. **If you are going to cheat, do it in less than one hour.** This prevents the insulin spike so you won't store belly fat.

6. **No sugar.** Just stick to your 1–2 pieces of low-GI fruit per day. I promise you: you won't miss the sugar after a while. Also, you will lose weight and have more energy. That's great!

7. **Drink water. Lots!**

8. **No food three hours before bed.** When you don't eat then the glycogen (which is the sugar stored in your liver) is used for the next 6–8 hours. During this time, your body burns fat. You are actually burning fat while you sleep, and it's painless. Yahoo!

9. **Exercise.** *Please ...*

10. **Watch what you are saying to yourself.** Maintain a positive outlook and be hopeful.

"By altering our attitudes, we can alter our lives." – Zig Ziglar

"Be careful how you are talking to yourself, because you are listening." – Lisa M. Hayes

11. **Eat good fats.**

12. **Take your supplements.**

One last thought for you. I have given you the very best of my heart in this book. Now the goal is to incorporate it, to achieve your maximum energy with your best health.

You deserve all the applause, because all I've done is coach you. You are the true winners when you implement these principles into the lives of your family and yourself.

Your friend,

Isabel

References and Resources

Chapter One: Your Metabolism and Your Nutrition

1. Hyman, Dr. Mark. The Blood Sugar Solution. New York. Little, Brown and Co. 2012.
2. Rubin, Jordan. The Great Physician's Rx for Health and Wellness. Tennessee, Thomas Nelson Inc. 2005.
3. Foster, Helen. Easy GI Diet. London, Octopus Publishing Group Ltd. 2004.
4. Kessler, Dr. David. The End of Overeating: Taking Control of the Insatiable American Appetite. USA, Rodale Press. 2009.
5. Lundell, Dr. Dwight. Heart Surgeon Speaks Out on What Really Causes Heart Disease. Health Wellness Prevent Disease 01 March 2012.

Chapter Four: Why Winners Win

1. Hill, Napoleon. The Laws of Success in Sixteen Lessons. Conn. Ralston University Press. 2008.

Chapter Five: Sugar, Obesity and Our Future

1. Dufault R, et al. Mercury from chlor-alkali plants: measured concentrations in food product sugar. Environ Health. 2009 Jan 26;8:2
2. Bray GA, Nielsen SJ, Popkin BM. Consumption of high-fructose corn syrup in beverages may play a role in the epidemic of obesity. Am J Clin Nutr. 2004 Apr;79(4):537–43. Review.
3. Swithers SE, Davidson TL. A role for sweet taste: calorie predictive relations in energy regulation by rats. Behav Neurosci. 2008;122 (1):161–73.
4. Yang Q. Gain weight by "going diet?" Artificial sweeteners, and the neurobiology of sugar cravings. Yale J Biol Med. 2010 June: 83(2):101–108.
5. Lenoir M, et al. Intense sweetness surpasses cocaine reward. PLoS One. 2007;2 (1):e698.
6. Ludwig DS. Artificially sweetened beverages: cause for concern. JAMA.2009 Dec 9;302 (22):2477–78.
7. http://apps.nccd.cdc.gov/DDTSTRS/FactSheet.aspx (National Diabetes Fact 2007).

Chapter Seven: Putting It All Together

1. Gaby AR. Nutritional Interventions for Muscle Cramps. Integrative Medicine 2007/8, 6(6):20–23.

2. Rossier P, van Erven S, Wade DT. The effect of magnesium oral therapy on spasticity in a patient with multiple sclerosis. European Journal of Neurology 2000, 7(6): 741–744.

3. Braun L & Cohen M, Chromium, Herbs and Natural Supplements: An evidence-based guide 3rd Edition Sydney, Elsevier, 2010, pp. 320–326.

4. Facchinetti F, et al, Magnesium prophylaxis of menstrual migraine: effects on intracellular magnesium Headache, 1991: 31:298–301.

5. Peikert A, et al, Prophylaxis of migraine with oral magnesium: results from a prospective, multi-center, placebo-controlled and double-blind randomized study. Cephalalgia, 196:16:257–263.

6. Sun-Edelstein C and Mauskop A. Role of magnesium in the pathogenesis and treatment of migraine. Expert Review of Neurotherapeutics, 2009; 9(3):369.

7. Braun L, Cohen M. Zinc, Herbs and Natural Supplements; an evidence based guide; Elsevier Australia 2010, pp. 1037–1054.

8. Braun L, Cohen M. Selenium-Herbs, and Natural Supplements; an evidence based guide; Elsevier Australia 2010, pp. 844–56.

9. Butterworth R. Chapter 23: Thiamine. In Shils ME, et al (Eds), Modern Nutrition in Health and Disease 10th Edition, Philadelphia, Lippincott Williams and Wilkins 2006: pp. 426–433.

10. Homocysteine Lowering Trialists Collaboration. Dose-dependent effects of folic acid on blood concentrations of homocysteine: a meta analysis of the randomized trials. Am J Clin Nutr 2005; 82(4): 806–12.

11. Mark Hyman, MD . The Blood Sugar Solution, p.75–77.

12. Nikooyeh B, et al. Daily consumption of vitamin D- or vitamin D + calcium-fortified yogurt drink improved glycemin control in patients with type 2 diabetes: a randomized clinical trial. Am J Clin Nutr. 2011 Apr; 93(4):764–71.

13. Jennifer Bowden. The Vitamin D Factor, New Zealand Listener. April 21, 2012. Issue 3754.

14. Institute of Functional Medicine.

DIETARY SUPPLEMENT FACT SHEET

Vitamin D. Office of Dietary Supplements (ODS). National Institutes of Health (NIH). Retrieved 2010–04 11. b.Cedric F. Garland, Dr PH, FACE, Edward D. Gorham, MPH, PhD, Sharif B. Mohr, MPH, Frank C. Garland, PhD.

Vitamin D for cancer prevention: Global perspective. Annals of Epidemiology. Volume 19, Issue 7, Pages 468–483 (July 2009). c.P. Lips, D. Hosking, K. Lippuner, J. M. Norquist, L. Wehren, G. Maalouf, S. Ragi-Eis, J. Chandler.

The prevalence of vitamin D inadequacy amongst women with osteoporosis: an international epidemiological investigation. Volume 260, Issue 3, pages 245–254, September 2006 d.Siegfried Segaer.

Vitamin D regulation of cathelicidin in the skin: Toward a renaissance of vitamin D in Dermatology? Journal of Investigative Dermatology (2008) 128, 773–775. doi:10.1038/jid.2008.35 e. Plotnikoff GA, Quigley JM.

Prevalence of severe hypovitaminosis D in patients with persistent, nonspecific musculoskeletal pain. Mayo Clin Proc. 2003;78(12):1463–1470. f. Al Faraj, Saud MD; Al Mutairi, Khalaf MD.

Vitamin D deficiency and chronic low back pain in Saudi Arabia. Spine:15 January 2003 – Volume 28 – Issue 2 – pp 177–179. g.Armstrong, D.; Meenagh, G.; Bickle, I.; Lee, A.; Curran, E.; Finch, M

Vitamin D deficiency is associated with anxiety and depression in fibromyalgia. Clinical Rheumatology. Volume 26, Number 4, 551–554, DOI: 10.1007/s10067-006-0348-5 h. Mathieu C, Gysemans C, Giulietti A, Bouillon R.

Vitamin D and diabetes. Diabetologia. 2006 Jan;49(1):217–8. i. Mackay-Sim A, Féron F, Eyles D, Burne T, McGrath J. Schizophrenia, vitamin D, and brain development. Int Rev Neurobiol. 2004;59:351–80. j.

Vitamin D Deficiency Common in Patients with Chronic Migraine. *http://www.medscape. com/viewarticle/577151* k. Ginanjar E, Sumariyono, Setiati S, Setiyohadi B.

Vitamin D and autoimmune disease. Acta Med Indones. 2007 Jul–Sep;39(3):133–41. l. Lisa M. Bodnar, Janet M. Catov, Hyagriv N. Simhan, Michael F. Holick, Robert W. Powers and James M. Roberts.

Maternal vitamin D deficiency increases the risk of preeclampsia. The Journal of Clinical Endocrinology & Metabolism Vol. 92, No. 9 3517–3522 m.Int J Epidemiol. 1990 Sep;19(3):559–63.

Myocardial infarction is inversely associated with plasma 25-hydroxyvitamin D3 levels: a community-based study. Scragg R, Jackson R, Holdaway IM, Lim T, Beaglehole R. Department of Community Health, University of Auckland , New Zealand. n. Li YC, Kong J, Wei M, Chen ZF, Liu SQ, Cao LP.

1,25-Dihydroxyvitamin D(3) is a negative endocrine regulator of the renin-angiotensin system. J Clin Invest. 2002;110(2):229–238. o. Ramagopalan SV, Maugeri NJ, Handunnetthi L, Lincoln MR, Orton S-M, et al. (2009) Expression of the multiple sclerosis-associated MHC Class II Allele HLA-DRB1*1501 Is regulated by vitamin D. PLoS Genet 5(2): e1000369. doi:10.1371/ journal.pgen.1000369 p. Anderson L, Cotterchio M, Vieth R, Knight J.

Vitamin D and calcium intakes and breast cancer risk in pre- and postmenopausal women. Am J Clin Nutr 2010; 91(6): 1699–1701. q.Garland CF, Gorham ED, Mohr SB, et al.

Vitamin D and prevention of breast cancer: Pooled analysis. J Steroid Biochem Mol Biol 2007;103:708–11. r.Bruce W Hollis and Carol L Wagner.

Assessment of dietary vitamin D requirements during pregnancy and lactation. American Journal of Clinical Nutrition, Vol. 79, No. 5, 717–726, May 2004

About the Author

DR. ISABEL BERTRAN-HUNSINGER is a Cuban-American, now living in the North Island of New Zealand. She moved from the USA to NZ to offer the family a different way of life, and yes, she has gotten that. Her girls even have the gorgeous Kiwi accent. She loves to do anything that keeps her fitness going, and enjoys biking, walking, trekking and training at the gym. Her husband Michael and Isabel have been in love (yes, marriage!) for 33 years and are excited about reaching 100 years young, together. Isabel thoroughly loves her walk with God and says, "my Christianity is the backbone of my life."

Dr. Isabel believes that you are your own best doctor, you just need a health coach to guide you. The goal is to have fun while learning simple steps to nutritional literacy.

Dr. Isabel offers health coaching to clients all over the world. She currently has a limited number of spaces available for 1×1 consultations via Skype, or other media sources. Contact her via email or Skype to set up an initial consultation.

PLEASE NOTE: Dr. Isabel's role is not to replace your physician. Consultation with her as your Healthy Lifestyle Coach should take place alongside your doctor's advice to empower your health, so you can live 'Life to the Max'.

Isabel Bertran-Hunsinger M.D. (aka Dr. Isabel)

University Of Colorado Medical School 1991

Southern Colorado Family Practice Residency 1995

Fellow of the Royal New Zealand College of General Practice 2005

Member of the Institute of Functional Medicine

Dr. Isabel's speaking availability

Dr. Isabel is available to speak at corporate functions, business team-building, and public groups. *Reclaim Your Health Workshop* (Healthy Lifestyle Programme), would be an excellent way to improve productivity on a personal and business team level. We can provide personalised assessment programmes for you and your staff. A healthy team engages better around company goals, and team members are mentally present and focused. This leads to greater productivity, which leads to greater profitability. To have your team, or you personally, 'Living Life to the Max', give Dr. Isabel a call, Skype or e-mail today.

Whether you want a health coach, inspirational speaker, or guidance on natural supplements, Dr. Isabel can be contacted via Skype, Facebook, Twitter or email. Please refer to the details below:

Skype: *isabel.hunsinger*
Facebook: *www.facebook.com/doctoronamission*
Twitter: *www.twitter.com/purelifestyle1*
Website/Blog: *www.doctoronamission.com*

To be a member of the doctoronamission team, please join our Healthy Lifestyle Club at **www.doctoronamission.com**